DEDICATION

To my wife, Linda M. Sinatra, and our children, Kristen, Lauren, and Elizabeth.

— **RSS**

Surgeon's Guide to Postsurgical Pain Management: Colorectal and Abdominal Surgery

First Edition

Raymond S. Sinatra, MD, PhD
Professor Emeritus of Anesthesiology
Yale University School of Medicine

Sergio Larach, MD
The Center for Colon & Rectal Surgery
Orlando, FL

Sonia L. Ramamoorthy, MD
Assistant Professor in Residence
Department of Surgery
University of California, San Diego

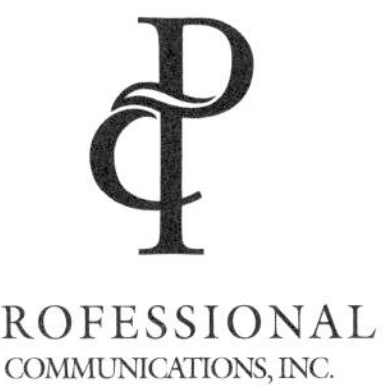

PROFESSIONAL
COMMUNICATIONS, INC.

Professional Communications, Inc.
A Medical Publishing & Communications Company

400 Center Bay Drive
West Islip, NY 11795
(t) 631/661-2852
(f) 631/661-2167

PO Box 10
Caddo, OK 74729-0010
(t) 580/367-9838
(f) 580/367-9989

For orders only, please call
1-800-337-9838
or visit our website at
www.pcibooks.com

ISBN: 978-1-932610-72-7

Printed in the United States of America

Disclaimer

The opinions expressed in this publication reflect those of the authors. However, the authors make no warranty regarding the contents of the publication. The protocols described herein are general and may not apply to a specific patient. Any product mentioned in this publication should be taken in accordance with the prescribing information provided by the manufacturer.

This text is printed on recycled paper. 

TABLE OF CONTENTS

TABLES

FIGURES

1

Current Management of Postsurgical Pain

by Raymond S. Sinatra MD, PhD

Introduction

Pain following surgery is among the most common of patient complaints encountered by surgeons and other health professionals, and it remains a major cause of patient dissatisfaction and delayed hospital discharge. With regard to surgical pain, there is certainly a lot of it about. There are approximately 73 million surgeries performed annually in the United States[1] and up to 70% of these patients experience pain postsurgery.[2-4] By 2005, the number of inpatient surgical procedures had risen to 26.6 million, with a large majority associated with moderate to very severe pain. The number of ambulatory surgical procedures appears to be increasing at an even greater rate, based on the current trend of increasing patient preference, increased use of laparoscopic procedures, and the rising number of ambulatory surgery centers.[2,5,6] Severe acute pain is the most common reason for admission to the emergency department (ED), and a large proportion of patients presenting with surgical- or trauma-related problems report pain of severe to very severe intensity.

Surgery involves highly invasive trespass of the human body in an effort to correct or control disease states and pathologic processes. Tissue dissection and associated inflammatory responses generate intense noxious stimulation, which, if poorly controlled, can result in:

- Hemodynamic instability
- Pulmonary dysfunction

- Impaired rehabilitation
- Development of persistent pain.

Optimal control of moderate to severe postsurgical pain is not only a basic human right[7] but can facilitate return to baseline functionality. Unfortunately, many caregivers have limited knowledge of opioid and nonopioid analgesic pharmacology and commonly underestimate postsurgical dose range while overestimating analgesic duration and risks of overdose.[8,9]

Current Standards of Analgesic Dosing

In recent years, caregivers and national societies have become increasingly aware of the importance of pain management, with the American Pain Society declaring the 10-year period beginning in 2001 as the "Decade of Pain."[10] The Joint Commission on Accreditation of Healthcare Organizations (JCAHO), also known as the Joint Commission, has mandated that pain intensity be measured regularly as the "Fifth Vital Sign" and that complaints of inadequate relief be treated promptly.[11]

The Agency for Healthcare Research and Quality and the Joint Commission have suggested that hospital performance standards include reductions in the incidence and severity of postsurgical pain and improvements in patient satisfaction and comfort.[12] Other organizations, including the International Association for the Study of Pain (IASP), American Society of Anesthesiologists (ASA), and the American Academy of Pain Medicine (AAPM), have also tried to address the problem of analgesic under-medication through evidence-based clinical practice guidelines and position statements designed to overcome deficiencies in analgesic delivery.[12] Rationales for providing effective pain control are presented in **Table 1.1**.

Significant efforts have been made to improve postsurgical pain management by providing physician

TABLE 1.1 — Why Should We Be So Concerned About Postsurgical Pain?

- There is always a humanitarian need to reduce pain and suffering.
- Poor pain control can adversely affect outcome in elderly and high-risk patients.
- Joint Commission and American Pain Society mandates underscore the importance of optimal pain management (pain as "Fifth Vital Sign").
- Patients are knowledgeable about new forms of therapy.
- Hospitals are being ranked on how well or how poorly they and their surgical staff manage pain.
- Hospitals are ranked according to the quality of pain management they provide.
- Hospitals and caregivers are increasingly liable for pain and suffering.

and patient education and increasing use of patient-controlled analgesia (PCA). Intravenous (IV) PCA was developed to overcome deficiencies associated with PRN intramuscular (IM) and IV analgesic dosing in which:

- Patients often wait too long to request pain relief.
- Staff may not be able to immediately deliver medication.
- Therapeutic plasma concentrations may not be uniformly maintained.[13]

A pain cycle characterized by alternating periods of oversedation and severe pain was a common occurrence and impacted ambulation and other measures of return to functionality (**Figure 1.1**).

With patient self-administration techniques, cycles of increasing pain and delays in analgesic administration may be eliminated, and patient satisfaction with therapy improves. Morphine is the most commonly prescribed opioid for PCA; however, hydromorphone appears to have a superior adverse-effect profile, and, in recent years, an increasing number of patients are treated with this agent.[14] Basal infusions or an hourly

FIGURE 1.1 — Patient Pain Cycle: PRN vs PCA Opioid Dosing

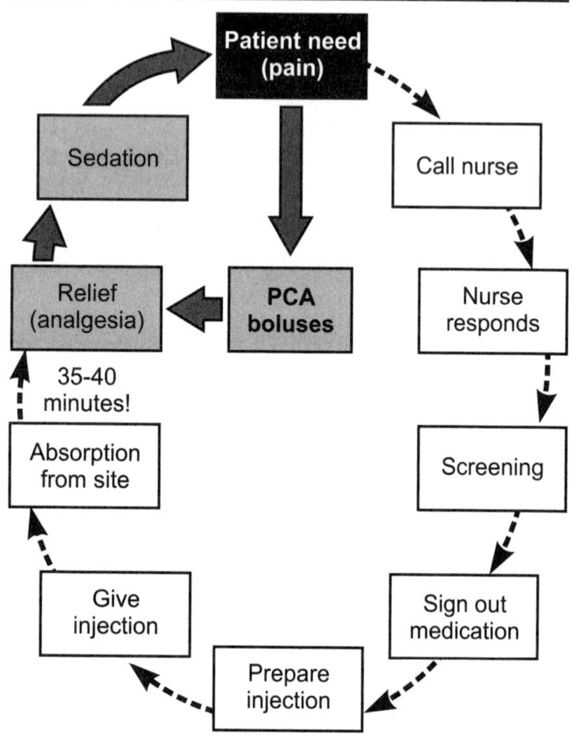

In a relative ranking of patient concerns, avoiding postoperative nausea and vomiting was the most important in this study.

Eberhart LH, et al. *Br J Anaesth*. 2002;89(5):760-761.

rate of opioid administration not controlled by the patient were originally advocated for severe pain or to improve sleep; such benefits have not been observed in controlled trials.[15] Moreover, basal infusions reduce the inherent safety of patient-initiated dosing. For this reason, basal infusion dosing should be restricted in dependent patients who require baseline opioids for a chronic pain condition in addition to that needed to control surgical pain.[16]

The major problem with IV-PCA is that "tethering" the patient to a large bulky device may impede ambulation, and prolonged duration of therapy results in increasing morbidity, including ileus and opioid-induced bowel dysfunction. For this reason, whenever possible, such therapy should be supplemented with nonopioid analgesics and neural blockade with local anesthetics. In addition, IV-PCA should be discontinued as soon as patients are able to tolerate oral analgesics (**Table 1.2**).

TABLE 1.2 — IV-PCA: Present-Day Application

- PCA should not be employed as monotherapy.
- Avoid high opioid-dose exposure and basal infusions.
- Discontinue as soon as the patient tolerates oral diet.
- PCA should be supplemented with continuous regional blockade and nonopioid adjuvants (30% to 80% reduction in morphine dose).
- PCA opioids may be combined with ketamine in patients with chronic pain and/or opioid dependency.

Many surgeons agree with the concept that analgesic intervention is most effective when made in advance of the pain stimulus rather than in reaction to it.[17] Many employ preemptive analgesia, including pre-incisional infiltration of local anesthetic and preoperative administration of nonsteroidal anti-inflammatory drugs (NSAIDs). Preemptive analgesic dosing has been shown to provide measurable reductions in pain following emergence from anesthesia and for the remainder of the postsurgical period. Reductions in pain intensity and opioid-sparing effects are generally superior to those observed when either NSAIDs or neural blockade with local anesthetics is provided following emergence from surgery. The major exception to preoperative analgesic dosing is observed with IV or oral opioids, which may initiate acute tolerance or hyperalgesic effects that can actually increase postsurgical pain intensity and opioid requirements.[18]

Multimodal Analgesia

Complete abolition of postsurgical pain (pain prevention) is difficult to achieve with a single drug or analgesic technique. In order to avoid dose-dependent adverse effects associated with reliance on one agent or technique, many surgeons employ "balanced" or multimodal analgesic regimens by which a variety of analgesics that work peripherally or in the central nervous system (CNS) may be administered in an effort to gain analgesic synergy and opioid dose-sparing effects.[19]

Multimodal strategies require additional caregiver knowledge regarding optimal dosing of each analgesic component, as well as skills in tissue infiltration and regional analgesia. The foundation of multimodal analgesia is peripheral neural blockade (PNB) and local anesthetic infiltration provided by the surgeon or the anesthesiology team. Recent advances in PNB, particularly the introduction of ultrasound guidance and stimulating catheters, has dramatically improved the reliability, acceptance, and use of this form of pain management. Peripheral local anesthetic blockade is particularly useful in patients who are expected to experience severe pain and for those who are highly sensitive to opioids. Techniques including wound-site local anesthetic infusion using gas-charged "Pain Buster" pumps, sciatic and femoral nerve block, and brachial plexus blockade can provide effective relief from extremely painful orthopedic, abdominal, and thoracic procedures. In addition, the recently FDA-approved local analgesic EXPAREL™ (bupivacaine liposome injectable suspension) will provide a more convenient alternative to complex elastomeric pumps and bags that are currently used to deliver local anesthetics over prolonged periods.

A 2006 meta-analysis of data from 19 randomized clinical trials evaluated the efficacy of continuous PNB with local anesthetics vs oral or parenteral opioid analgesia in 603 patients who had primarily undergone lower extremity surgery.[20] PNB provided better postsurgical analgesia (P<0.001) with significantly fewer gastrointestinal (GI) adverse effects compared with opioids alone. Other investigators[21] evaluated the efficacy of analgesia delivered by IV-PCA, continuous epidural infusion, or continuous 3-in-1 block following total knee arthroplasty (TKA). Continuous epidural infusion and continuous 3-in-1 block resulted in superior pain relief, fewer adverse effects, and faster knee rehabilitation compared with IV-PCA.

NSAID analgesics reduce pain and peripheral inflammation and are commonly prescribed. Oral celecoxib (Celebrex) and ibuprofen injection (Caldolor) are NSAID class drugs that are potentially safer than ketorolac (Toradol) and provide effective pain relief while reducing opioid dose requirements.[22] Both agents block cyclooxygenase (COX)-2, inhibiting prostaglandin synthesis following tissue injury but are less specific for COX-1, which maintains platelet function and gastric mucosal integrity. Injectable ibuprofen and celecoxib are contraindicated in patients with gastric bleeding and renal disease. A new preparation, IV acetaminophen, provides another multimodal option that reduces postsurgical pain and opioid dose with a high degree of safety.[23]

Preemptive and multimodal administration of these and other nonopioid analgesics is increasingly embraced and offers improved and more uniform analgesic effects than overreliance on potent short-duration opioids.

The Effectiveness of Current Pain Management

Despite the development of novel analgesics and analgesic techniques, the management of postsurgical pain remains inadequate across various treatment settings, with a substantial proportion of patients continuing to experience intense pain despite the availability of effective treatment.[2,24-26] Moderate-to-severe pain can persist for many days following hospital discharge. In a large study of ambulatory surgical patients, McGrath and colleagues[25] reported that >30% of patients reported moderate to severe pain scores on postsurgical day 1 (6.3 cm on a 0-10–cm VAS scale) and pain intensity decreased only slightly (5.6 cm) by postsurgical day 3 suggesting that current modalities do not adequately cover the prolonged postsurgical period where pain commonly occurs. Beauregard and coworkers[26] assessed pain in patients recovering from ambulatory surgery and found that 40% of patients reported moderate to severe pain during the first 24 hours after discharge; pain decreased over time but was severe enough to interfere with daily activities and with return to work for several days to weeks postsurgery.

Several well-controlled and highly regarded epidemiologic investigations employed telephone questionnaires and patient surveys to assess pain intensity and satisfaction with therapy in patients who had undergone surgery in teaching hospitals or community hospitals.[2,24] In an initial study performed in 1994, Warfield and Kahn[24] found that approximately 75% of patients experienced pain after surgery and of those, 80% rated their pain as moderate to extreme. In a follow-up study performed in 2003, Apfelbaum and coworkers[2] evaluated the effectiveness of pain management immediately following major surgery until 2 weeks after discharge. Two hundred fifty patients were asked to assess the severity of pain, satisfaction with pain medication, education provided by caregivers, and perceptions about postsurgical pain and pain medications. Approximately 80% of patients experienced pain during the evaluation interval, and the majority (86%) classified their pain as moderate, severe, or extreme.[24]

The lack of pain-intensity differences between two similar trials performed approximately 8 years apart is strikingly similar (**Figure 1.2**), as well as discouraging. It is likely that identical patient surveys performed today would reveal similar number of patients reporting severe or very severe pain-intensity scores and no

FIGURE 1.2 — **Despite Improvements in Analgesic Therapy and Delivery, Patients Continue to Experience Moderate-to-Severe Postsurgical Pain**[a]

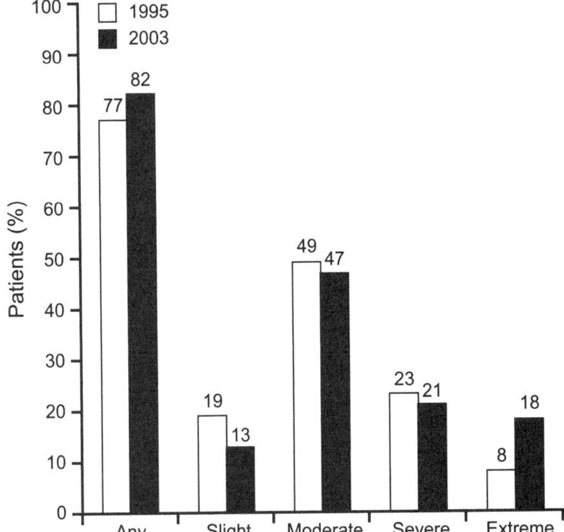

[a] Pain experienced after surgery until 2 weeks postdischarge.

Warfield CA, Kahn CH. *Anesthesiology*. 1995;83(5):1090-1094; Apfelbaum JL, et al. *Anesth Analg*. 2003;97(2):534-540.

overall improvement in postsurgical pain management. Thus there is a critical need for further improvement in analgesic therapy, particularly in high-risk settings where severe to very severe pain is associated with increased cardiovascular and pulmonary complications as well as delays in hospital discharge and rehabilitation.

A number of factors have been identified that contribute to inadequate postsurgical pain management, including:

- Surgeon- and patient-related misconceptions regarding opioid use
- Overreliance on opioid analgesics (opioid monotherapy)

- Side effects
- Patient noncompliance with analgesic therapy
- Inadequate patient assessment
- Technology-related failures (*see Chapter 2*).

While a new epidemiologic survey has yet to be performed, a follow-up study is currently in development and it is highly unlikely that pain intensity will have improved to any great extent during the decade following these reports.[2,24]

Cost-Related Consequences of Poorly Controlled Pain

Poorly controlled postsurgical pain has consequences beyond the immediate perception of pain and can negatively impact patients' well-being on multiple levels.

■ Diminished Patient Functioning

Patients who had undergone radical prostatectomy, total hip replacement, or total knee replacement were assessed for pain, health-related quality of life, and physical and social functioning at 4 weeks post–hospital discharge using the Short Form (SF)-36 quality-of-life questionnaire. Patients in each surgical group demonstrated significant alterations from baseline scores, including increased bodily pain and diminished social functioning, quality of sleep, and ability to perform physical activities.[27] Dihle and colleagues[28] studied the relationship between pain intensity and sleep disturbance in 77 patients following joint replacement surgery. Sleep was most affected in patients with severe pain (numeric rating score 6 to 10) compared with those with mild pain (score 1 to 3) or moderate pain (score 4 to 5) on the third day after surgery ($P < 0.02$). Severe pain also significantly impaired a range of other functions, including walking ability, general activity, social relationships, and mood.

■ Longer Hospital Stays

Postsurgical pain also results in increased resource utilization and health care costs. For example, Morrison and colleagues[29] studied 411 patients undergoing surgical repair of a hip fracture and reported that patients with higher postsurgical pain scores had significantly longer hospital length of stay (LOS), were significantly less likely to be ambulating by postsurgical day 3, took significantly longer to ambulate further than a bedside chair, and had significantly lower locomotion scores at 6 months.

■ Hospital Readmission

Poorly controlled pain is one of the most common reasons for postsurgical hospital readmission following ambulatory surgery and may substantially increase the cost of hospital care. In a study of 20,817 patients recovering from same-day surgery, over one third (38%) of the 313 patients who returned to the hospital reported pain as the main reason for their readmission.[30] The average cost per patient for readmission due to pain was $1869 per visit (**Table 1.3**). Given that >80% of patients experience postsurgical pain despite the availability of effective analgesics, inadequate postsurgical pain relief will continue to add to the

TABLE 1.3 — Poorly Controlled Pain After Ambulatory Surgery: Mean Cost of Follow-Up Care

Parameter	*N*	Mean Cost Per Patient (USD)[a]
All pain unanticipated admissions or readmissions	117	$1869
Emergency department visits	109	$986
Non–pain-related readmissions	8	$13,902

[a] Based on cost of care in 1999.

Coley KC, et al. *J Clin Anesth*. 2002;14(5):349-353.

already high economic burden of treatment by extending recovery time and hospital LOS.

■ Development of Chronic Pain Syndrome

A final and often unrecognized risk associated with undertreatment of postsurgical pain is the development of persistent pain. An estimated 10% to 50% of patients undergoing operations such as leg amputation, coronary bypass surgery, breast surgery, and groin hernia repair later develop persistent pain.[31] The primary predictor for development of chronic pain syndrome is the intensity of acute postsurgical pain.[32] Collectively, these data underscore the importance of prompt and effective pain management for improving quality of life and minimizing patient morbidity, not only in the period immediately following the acute pain episode but possibly throughout the remainder of the patient's life.

Thus it is extremely important to identify and prioritize patients at risk for experiencing very severe pain postsurgery and to meet with anesthesiology and nursing caregivers to develop an analgesic plan appropriately tailored to meet patient needs.[33] This may include a continuous epidural block, which when initiated prior to incision has been shown to significantly reduce the incidence of persistent pain states 12 months following surgery.[34] The role of continuous neural blockade and certain analgesics (eg, ketamine, gabapentin, local anesthetics, clonidine) in reducing the incidence of persistent pain is still unknown.

Cost-Related Consequences of Opioid-Related Adverse Events

Opioid-related adverse events are relatively common and many clinicians consider them simply part of the cost of providing, or attempting to provide, adequate pain control. In the 2-week period following a patient's surgery, 50% of patients report nausea and/or vomiting, 41% who receive an opioid report drowsiness, 26% report constipation, 10% report itching, and 8% report difficulty urinating.[35]

Mostly due to underreporting of hospital-acquired adverse events, the exact frequency of opioid-related adverse events in the postsurgical setting is largely unknown.[36] A recent retrospective study evaluating administrative data from 324,568 patients who underwent common surgical procedures (eg, hip replacement, laparoscopic cholecystectomy, laparoscopic colectomy, open colectomy, and total abdominal hysterectomy) at 381 US hospitals demonstrated that at least 20% of these patients had documentation supporting the occurrence of an opioid-related adverse event during their hospital course.[37]

In another study evaluating total cost and LOS outliers in 3654 patients who underwent abdominal hysterectomy, the equianalgesic opioid load in outliers was twice the load seen in controls (12% v 1%; $P<0.01$) and respiratory adverse events were 12-fold more common in outliers than in controls ($P<0.01$), with a more than 2-fold increase in GI adverse effects (44% vs 19%; $P<0.01$). A comparison of total cost for admission between outliers and controls demonstrated significantly higher costs in the outlier group ($14,275 vs $5745), in which total opioid consumption was more than double that of the control group (150 mg vs 74 mg; $P<0.01$) and respiratory- and GI-related opioid adverse events were significantly more common.[38]

■ Postoperative Ileus

Postoperative ileus (POI) is a predictable delay in GI motility that occurs after abdominal surgery and is well known to be exacerbated by opioids. When administered in doses adequate for human analgesia, morphine increases intestinal tone and contraction amplitude but mitigates propulsion in the colon. The net effect is diminished GI motility.[39] POI is associated with a greater incidence of postsurgical morbidity and is a common reason for increased LOS or readmission.[40-42]

An analysis of a large national database revealed that patients with coded POI experienced an increase in LOS (an additional 6 days) and higher health care costs (an additional $9417) per hospital stay compared with patients without coded POI.[43] In another study, Simons and colleagues utilized a large US managed-care database to retrospectively examine the magnitude and impact of GI and other opioid-related adverse events, as well as associated outcomes (eg, cost, LOS), in a surgical population.[44] Among 80% of 2,685,854 eligible patients who received an opioid during their hospital stay, GI-related adverse events were significantly associated with opioid use, even after eliminating effects of other factors that may result in the same adverse events. Opioid use was associated with an increased risk of 13 prespecified adverse events, with POI having the highest odds ratio. The adjusted mean increases in LOS and total costs for patients who experienced POI were 1.86 days and $4786, respectively.[44]

■ Central Nervous System

Combined CNS effects are known to account for the second highest percentage (30.3%) of evaluated opioid-related adverse events. Sedation and somnolence are the most commonly reported effects, with the latter ranging from <2% to >90% for various opioids and routes of administration.[45]

Literature from the past decade contains numerous case reports linking opioids to hallucinations, nightmares, and other CNS adverse events during the acute postsurgical period. Drug-associated psychoses, sleep impairment, dizziness, and somnolence were documented infrequently and inconsistently and in only a few reports. Meperidine and hydromorphone have been most commonly associated with adverse CNS events.[45]

Opioid-induced delirium, especially in the elderly, is of special concern. One study described delirium in nearly half of patients who received fentanyl for analgesia after bilateral knee replacement surgery. Postoperative delirium (POD), among the most common postsurgical complications in older patients, is associated with increased morbidity, mortality, LOS, and likelihood of nursing home placement.[46] As a result, POD contributes substantially to health care costs. Preoperative predictors of POD include age >70 years, preexisting cognitive impairment, history of alcohol abuse, depression, dehydration, visual impairment, and preoperative use of opiates. Postsurgical pain and certain medications (eg, meperidine, anticholinergics, benzodiazepines) are also associated with an increased risk of POD.[47]

■ Respiratory Depression

Respiratory depressive effects (due to inhibition of brain stem respiratory centers) are the least commonly reported of opioid-related adverse events. Nevertheless, they comprise the majority of severe opioid adverse outcome reports. Observational studies report a range in the occurrence of respiratory depression from 0.01% to 3.0%, an incidence that does not differ between single-injection neuraxial opioids and parenteral (ie, IV, IM, IV patient controlled) opioids. The incidence of respiratory depression does tend to increase in association with parenteral vs continuous epidural, epidural morphine or hydromorphone vs epidural fentanyl or sufentanil, higher vs lower opioid doses, and addition of parenteral opioids or hypnotics to neuraxial opioids.[48]

■ Urinary Retention

Approximately 18% of patients have been reported to have some form of urinary retention in cases when urinary function was recorded; the incidence is highest (30%) with intrathecal opioid administration, particularly with morphine. Urinary retention is primarily treated with catheterization, which may lead to complications such as hemorrhage, infection, and perforation, plus associated increased costs.[45]

■ Overall Hospital Costs

The occurrence of opioid-related adverse events following surgery creates a significant economic burden on health care providers.[49-52] In a retrospective study examining the financial impact of opioid-related adverse events, Oderda and colleagues found that patients experiencing opioid-related adverse events had a 7.4% increase in median total hospital costs and a 10.3% increase in median LOS.[53] In a similar study by Oderda and colleagues, surgical patients who experienced opioid-related adverse events had statistically significant increases in LOS (0.53 days) and in log-transformed cost (16%). The estimated log cost difference of 16%, if applied to the median cost/ patient in the nonadverse event group, averaged $840.[54]

After matching for age and severity of illness, a 2011 study by Oderda and associates[37] compared 62,814 surgical patients who experienced an opioid-related adverse event with 261,754 patients who did not have an opioid-related adverse event and demonstrated a significantly higher percentage of LOS and total cost outliers in the opioid-related adverse event group compared with the no opioid-related adverse event group (LOS: 13% vs 7% (P<0.0001) and total cost 8.0% vs 5.0% (P<0.0001), respectively. Patients with opioid-related adverse events had a 2.1 times higher likelihood (95% CI 2.1-2.2) of being a LOS outlier and a 1.4 times higher likelihood (95% CI 1.3-1.4) of being a cost outlier compared with patients who did not experience an opioid-related adverse event. The financial impact of any opioid-related adverse event was an additional $1030 and a 1.1 day LOS (**Figure 1.3** and **Figure 1.4**).

An analysis from a large health system in the northeastern United States comprised of six major medical centers suggests that total opioid burden and opioid-related adverse events may be responsible for extended LOSs and total cost among patients undergoing total abdominal hysterectomy (TAH). Outliers were defined as patients with the longest LOSs (5+ days). Opioid-related adverse events (respiratory and GI) were significantly more common in the outlier group. Outlier patients received twice as much opioid (in terms of IV morphine) as the controls and 92%

FIGURE 1.3 — Mean Outcomes (Total Cost/ Length of Stay) of Unmatched and Matched[a] Individuals With Common Surgeries[b] Comparing Opioid ADE With No-Opioid ADE

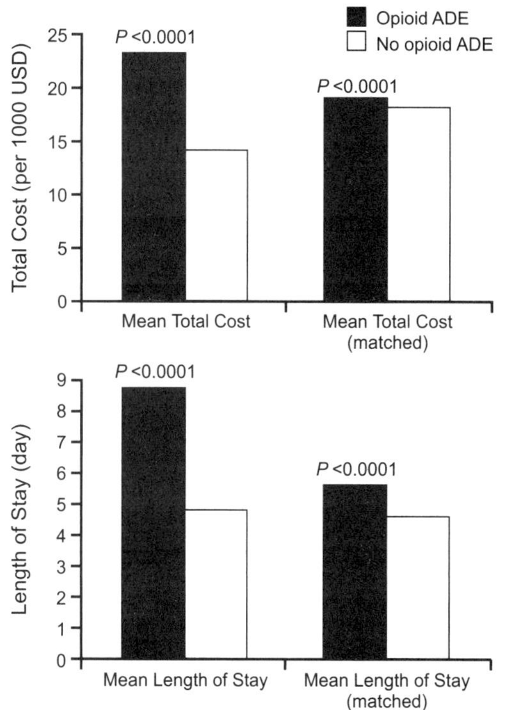

[a] Matched 1:3 where possible on age +/- 3 years, gender, and severity of illness.

[b] Hip replacement, laparoscopic cholescystectomy, laparoscopic colectomy, open colectomy, total abdominal hysterectomy.

Oderda G, et al. Poster presented at: 46th ASHP Midyear Clinical Meeting and Exhibition; December 4-8, 2011; New Orleans, LA. Poster 3-185.

FIGURE 1.4 — Matched[a] Adjusted[b] Odds Ratio of Being an Outlier With Common Surgeries[c] Comparing Opioid ADE With No-Opioid ADE

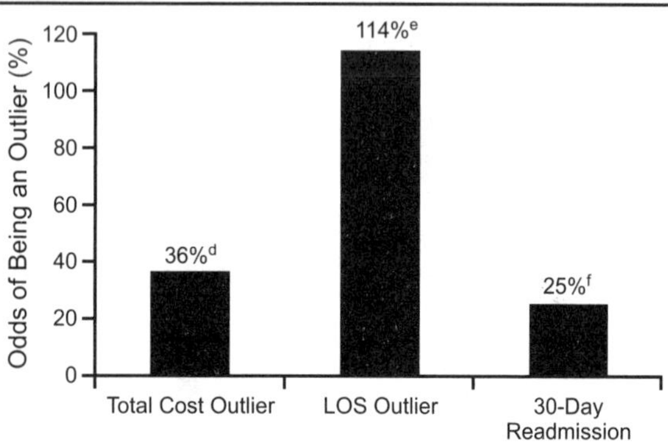

[a] Matched 1:3 where possible on age ± 3 years/gender/severity of illness.
[b] Adjusted for race/ethnicity, urbanicity, teaching status of hospital, geographic location, use of other analgesics.
[c] Hip replacement, laparoscopic cholecystectomy, laparoscopic colectomy, open colectomy, total abdominal hysterectomy.
[d] 95% CI, 1.30-1.44. Significant at the 0.05 level
[e] 95% CI, 2.06-2.22. Significant at the 0.05 level.
[f] 95% CI, 1.21-1.29. Significant at the 0.05 level.

Oderda G, et al. Poster presented at: 46th ASHP Midyear Clinical Meeting and Exhibition; December 4-8, 2011; New Orleans, LA. Poster 3-185.

and 91% of respiratory and GI opioid-related adverse events, respectively, occurred within 72 hours of leaving the operating room.[37]

Pain Management Performance Standards

Despite the pathophysiologic and pharmacoeconomic evidence presented here, many surgeons continue to question the need for improving postsurgical pain management, suggesting that acute pain is a necessary physiologic response to traumatic injury that will progressively diminish in intensity and eventually resolve. Most hospital administrators and reviewing organizations disagree, stating that optimal pain relief is a patient's right and that undermedication of pain is associated with significant morbidity and delay in return to baseline functionality (**Table 1.1**).

Data collected from local and regional patient-satisfaction surveys, including information sent to The Hospital Consumer Assessment of Healthcare Providers and Systems (HCAHPS), are increasingly being utilized to develop hospital performance standards for health care facilities.[55] The overall quality of pain management provided at each facility and by medical and surgical specialists affiliated with those institutions has become a key performance marker. Surveys focused on patient satisfaction with pain management may be used to rank health care facilities as best or worst, depending upon how well their patients' pain is controlled. Facilities where pain was "sometimes" or "never" well controlled have been ranked as worst. These rankings are presently published online or by US World Report rankings of hospital performance. It was no surprise that some hospitals were ranked far superior to others.[56] Patients are increasingly making decisions to select one facility over a nearby competitor, and superiority in providing pain management may influence their choice.

Postsurgical pain has become an increasingly important outcome impacting hospital quality measures and reimbursement. The Hospital Consumer Assessment of Healthcare Providers and Systems (HCAHPS) survey is the first national, standardized, publicly reported survey measuring and comparing patients' pain perceptions during their hospital experiences. In two 1-year, nationwide HCAHPS surveys of 3765 reporting hospitals conducted in 2008 and 2009, pain management received an average score of 68 (out of a possible 100), revealing much room for improvement.

Upcoming value-based purchasing mandates from the Center for Medicare and Medicaid Services (CMS) that utilize HCAHPS data will even further utilize pain measures as an important factor that will drive reimbursement and force hospitals to compete for improved patient-satisfaction scores that in turn will drive financial incentives. Inadequate control of postsurgical pain has negative consequences, which may cause decreased patient satisfaction, extended LOS, and readmissions, all of which increase overall costs. Hospital readmissions have recently garnered significant attention in the health care community since the passage of the Affordable Care Act in 2010. The new health law calls on the CMS to start measuring 30-day hospital readmission rates and to penalize poor performers. In October 2012, hospitals with high readmission rates will face penalties of 1% of their total Medicare billing with penalties increasing to 2% the following year. In a retrospective study in 20,817 same-day surgery patients, inadequate pain control was the most common reason (36%) for unplanned hospital admissions within the first 30 days following discharge. The mean charge per unanticipated admission or readmission due to pain was $1869 +/- $4553.[57]

Computerized surveillance of inpatient records may provide rapid identification of rare yet potentially serious opioid adverse events. By targeting perioperative administration of naloxone, employing computerized surveillance of patient records, pharmacists at Duke were able to detect cases of opioid-related oversedation and respiratory depression and correlate the extent of harm and associated medical costs associated with these events.[58] While serious events were rare (1.89 adverse drug events/1000 surgical cases), they tended to occur in high frequency in selected patients. Eleven of 69 serious events occurred in patients who had prior histories of harmful opioid-related oversedation. Such patients who experienced multiple events and are at increased risk for becoming LOS and cost outliers are particularly relevant to future studies seeking risk factors for opioid-induced respiratory depression or patients with significant alterations in hospital stay or cost of treatment related to treatment with IV and orally administered opioid analgesics.

The 2011 study by Oderda and associates of a large group of postsurgical patients experiencing an opioid-related adverse event demonstrated that opioid adverse events have a significant impact on prolonging hospital LOS and driving up total hospital costs associated with outliers. The results are instructive for surgeons and administrators alike and demonstrate that the costs associated with opioids and opioid-related adverse events are so significant that changes in analgesic treatment plans that embrace more expensive neural blockade techniques and nonopioid analgesic alternatives, including newer longer-acting local analgesics, should be considered for specific patient populations and surgical procedures.

The chapters that follow will present additional evidence that unrelieved postsurgical pain has consequences beyond satisfaction and can negatively impact patient well-being at multiple levels and lead to pain persistence. Chapters will also introduce existing, new, and emerging analgesics and dosing guidelines for specific populations that may be employed to optimally control postsurgical pain.

REFERENCES

1. Hutchison RW. Challenges in acute post-operative pain management. *Am J Health Syst Pharm*. 2007;64(6 suppl 4):S2-S5.
2. Apfelbaum JL, Chen C, Mehta SS, Gan TJ. Postoperative pain experience: results from a national survey suggest postoperative pain continues to be undermanaged. *Anesth Analg*. 2003;97(2):534-540.
3. Schug SA, Large RG. Economic considerations in pain management. *Pharmacoeconomics*. 1993;3(4):260-267.
4. Owen H, McMillan V, Rogowski D. Postoperative pain therapy: a survey of patients' expectations and their experiences. *Pain*. 1990;41(3):303-307.
5. DeFrances CJ, Cullen KA, Kozak LJ. National Hospital Discharge Survey: 2005 annual summary with detailed diagnosis and procedure data. *Vital Health Stat 13*. 2007;(165):1-209.
6. Bian J, Morrisey MA. Free-standing ambulatory surgery centers and hospital surgery volume. *Inquiry*. 2007;44(2):200-210.
7. Brennan F, Carr DB, Cousins M. Pain management: a fundamental human right. *Anesth Analg*. 2007;105(1):205-221.
8. Juhl IU, Christensen BV, Bülow HH, Wilbek H, Dreijer NC, Egelund B. Postoperative pain relief, from the patients' and the nurses' point of view. *Acta Anaesthesiol Scand*. 1993;37 (4):404-409.
9. Guru V, Dubinsky I. The patient vs. caregiver perception of acute pain in the emergency department. *J Emerg Med*. 2000; 18(1):7-12.
10. Gordon DB, Dahl JL, Miaskowski C, et al. American pain society recommendations for improving the quality of acute and cancer pain management: American Pain Society Quality of Care Task Force. *Arch Intern Med*. 2005;165(14):1574-1580.
11. Joint Commission on Accreditation of Healthcare Organizations. JCAHO Standards for Pain Management [referenced from the Comprehensive Accreditation Manual for Hospitals, Update 3, 1999 (effective January 1, 2001)]. Available at http://www.jointcommission.org/assets/1/18/Pain_Management.pdf. Accessed December 1, 2011.
12. Wells N, Pasero C, McCaffery M. Improving the quality of care through pain assessment and management. In: Hughes RG, ed. *Patient Safety and Quality: An Evidence-Based Handbook for Nurses*. Rockville, MD; Agency for Healthcare Research and Quality; 2008:469-497. http://www.ncbi.nlm.nih.gov/books/NBK2658. Accessed November 17 2011.

13. Chumbley GM, Hall GM, Salmon P. Why do patients feel positive about patient-controlled analgesia? *Anaesthesia*. 1999;54(4):386-389.

14. Rapp SE, Egan KJ, Ross BK, Wild LM, Terman GW, Ching JM. A multidimensional comparison of morphine and hydromorphone patient-controlled analgesia. *Anesth Analg*. 1996;82(5):1043-1048.

15. Sherman B, Enu I, Sinatra RS. PCA and other analgesic delivery systems. In: Sinatra RS, Viscusi G, DeLeon-Cassasola O, Ginsberg B, eds. *Acute Pain Management*. New York, NY: Cambridge Press; 2008.

16. Sinatra RS, Torres J, Bustos AM. Pain management after major orthopaedic surgery: current strategies and new concepts. *J Am Acad Orthop Surg*. 2002;10(2):117-129.

17. Woolf CJ, Chong MS. Preemptive analgesia--treating postoperative pain by preventing the establishment of central sensitization. *Anesth Analg*. 1993;77(2):362-379.

18. Angst MS, Clark JD. Opioid-induced hyperalgesia: a qualitative systematic review. *Anesthesiology*. 2006;104(3):570-587.

19. Buvanendran A, Kroin JS. Useful adjuvants for postoperative pain management. *Best Pract Res Clin Anaesthesiol*. 2007;21(1):31-49.

20. Richman JM, Liu SS, Courpas G, et al. Does continuous peripheral nerve block provide superior pain control to opioids? A meta-analysis. *Anesth Analg*. 2006;102(1):248-257.

21. Capdevila X, Barthelet Y, Biboulet P, Ryckwaert Y, Rubenovitch J, d'Athis F. Effects of perioperative analgesic technique on the surgical outcome and duration of rehabilitation after major knee surgery. *Anesthesiology*. 1999;91(1):8-15.

22. Southworth S, Peters J, Rock A, Pavliv L. A multicenter, randomized, double-blind, placebo-controlled trial of intravenous ibuprofen 400 and 800 mg every 6 hours in the management of postoperative pain. *Clin Ther*. 2009;31(9):1922-1935.

23. Sinatra RS, Jahr JS, Reynolds LW, Viscusi ER, Groudine SB, Payen-Champenois C. Efficacy and safety of single and repeated administration of 1 gram intravenous acetaminophen injection (paracetamol) for pain management after major orthopedic surgery. *Anesthesiology*. 2005;102(4):822-831.

24. Warfield CA, Kahn CH. Acute pain management. Programs in U.S. hospitals and experiences and attitudes among U.S. adults. *Anesthesiology*. 1995;83(5):1090-1094.

25. McGrath B, Elgendy H, Chung F, Kamming D, Curti B, King S. Thirty percent of patients have moderate to severe pain 24 hr after ambulatory surgery: a survey of 5,703 patients. *Can J Anaesth*. 2004;51(9):886-891.

26. Beauregard L, Pomp A, Choinière M. Severity and impact of pain after day-surgery. *Can J Anaesth*. 1998;45(4):304-311.

27. Strassels SA, McNicol E, Wagner AK, Rogers WH, Gouveia WA, Carr DB. Persistent postoperative pain, health-related quality of life, and functioning 1 month after hospital discharge. *Acute Pain*. 2004;6(3):95-104.

28. Dihle A, Helseth S, Kongsgaard UE, Paul SM, Miaskowski C. Using the American Pain Society's patient outcome questionnaire to evaluate the quality of postoperative pain management in a sample of Norwegian patients. *J Pain*. 2006;7(4):272-280.

29. Morrison RS, Magaziner J, McLaughlin MA, et al. The impact of post-operative pain on outcomes following hip fracture. *Pain*. 2003;103(3):303-311.

30. Coley KC, Williams BA, DaPos SV, Chen C, Smith RB. Retrospective evaluation of unanticipated admissions and readmissions after same day surgery and associated costs. *J Clin Anesth*. 2002;14(5):349-353.

31. Kehlet H, Jensen TS, Woolf CJ. Persistent postsurgical pain: risk factors and prevention. *Lancet*. 2006;367(9522):1618-1625.

32. Pluijms WA, Steegers MA, Verhagen AF, Scheffer GJ, Wilder-Smith OH. Chronic post-thoracotomy pain: a retrospective study. *Acta Anaesthesiol Scand*. 2006;50(7):804-808.

33. Vickers A, Bali S, Baxter A, et al. Consensus statement on the anticipation and prevention of acute postoperative pain: multidisciplinary RADAR approach. *Curr Med Res Opin*. 2009; 25(10):2557-2569.

34. Bach S, Noreng MF, Tjéllden NU. Phantom limb pain in amputees during the first 12 months following limb amputation, after preoperative lumbar epidural blockade. *Pain*. 1988;33(3):297-301.

35. Apfelbaum JL, Chen C, Mehta SS, Gan TJ. Postoperative pain experience: results from a national survey suggest postoperative pain continues to be undermanaged. *Anesth Analg*. 2003;97(2):534-540.

36. Classen DC, Resar R, Griffin F, et al. 'Global trigger tool' shows that adverse events in hospitals may be ten times greater than previously measured. *Health Aff (Millwood)*. 2011;30(4):581-589.

37. Oderda GM, Gan TJ, Robinson SB, Johnson B. Opioid-related adverse events increase length of stay and drive up total cost of care in a national database of postsurgical patients. Poster presented at: 46th ASHP Midyear Clinical Meeting and Exhibition; December 4-8, 2011; New Orleans, LA. Poster 3-185.

38. Moleski R, Adamson R, Lew I. Cost and quality implications of opioid-based post surgical pain control in total abdominal hysterectomy: a study of cost outliers and opioid related adverse events. Poster presented at: 46th ASHP Midyear Clinical Meeting and Exhibition; December 4-8, 2011; New Orleans, LA. Poster 3-192.

39. Carroll J, Alavi K. Pathogenesis and management of postoperative ileus. *Clin Colon Rectal Surg*. 2009;22(1):47-50.

40. Chang SS, Baumgartner RG, Wells N, Cookson MS, Smith JA Jr. Causes of increased hospital stay after radical cystectomy in a clinical pathway setting. *J Urol*. 2002;167(1):208-211.

41. Kariv Y, Wang W, Senagore AJ, Hammel JP, Fazio VW, Delaney CP. Multivariable analysis of factors associated with hospital readmission after intestinal surgery. *Am J Surg*. 2006;191(3):364-371.

42. Delaney CP, Senagore AJ, Viscusi ER, et al. Postoperative upper and lower gastrointestinal recovery and gastrointestinal morbidity in patients undergoing bowel resection: pooled analysis of placebo data from 3 randomized controlled trials. *Am J Surg*. 2006;191(3):315-319.

43. Hutchison RW, Chon EH, Tucker WF, Gilder R, Moss J, Daniel P. A comparison of a fentanyl, morphine, and hydromorphone patient-controlled intravenous delivery for acute postoperative analgesia: a multicenter study of opioid-induced adverse reactions. *Hosp Pharm*. 2006;41:659-663.

44. Simons R, Kim M, Chow W. Retrospective analyses of adverse events and economic costs. Regional Anesthesia and Pain Medicine 2009; Poster Session 3: Abstract 17.

45. Wheeler M, Oderda GM, Ashburn MA, Lipman AG. Adverse events associated with postoperative opioid analgesia: a systematic review. *J Pain*. 2002;3(3):159-180.

46. Jankowski CJ. Delirium and postoperative cognitive dysfunction. In: Sieber FE, ed. *Geriatric Anesthesia*. New York, NY: McGraw-Hill; 2007:267-279.

47. Robinson TN, Raeburn CD, Tran ZV, Angles EM, Brenner LA, Moss M. Postoperative delirium in the elderly: risk factors and outcomes. *Ann Surg*. 2009;249(1):173-178.

48. American Society of Anesthesiologists Task Force on Neuraxial Opioids; Horlocker TT, Burton AW, Connis RT, et al. Practice guidelines for the prevention, detection, and management of respiratory depression associated with neuraxial opioid administration. *Anesthesiology*. 2009;110(2):218-230.

49. Hill RP, Lubarsky DA, Phillips-Bute B, et al. Cost-effectiveness of prophylactic antiemetic therapy with ondansetron, droperidol, or placebo. *Anesthesiology*. 2000;92(4):958-967.

50. Kovac AL. Prevention and treatment of postoperative nausea and vomiting. *Drugs*. 2000;59(2):213-243.

51. Watcha MF, Smith I. Cost-effectiveness analysis of antiemetic therapy for ambulatory surgery. *J Clin Anesth*. 1994;6(5):370-377.

52. White PF. Management of postoperative pain and emesis. *Can J Anaesth*. 1995;42(11):1053-1055.

53. Oderda GM, Said Q, Evans RS, et al. Opioid-related adverse drug events in surgical hospitalizations: impact on costs and length of stay. *Ann Pharmacother*. 2007;41(3):400-406.

54. Oderda GM, Evans RS, Lloyd J, et al. Cost of opioid-related adverse drug events in surgical patients. *J Pain Symptom Manage*. 2003;25(3):276-283.

55. US Department of Health and Human Services, Centers for Medicare and Medicaid. HCAHPS: Patients' Perspectives of Care Survey. http://www.cms.gov/HospitalQualityInits/30_HospitalHCAHPS.asp. Accessed December 1, 2011.

56. US World Report rankings of pain management at major hospitals in the United States. http://health.usnews.com/health-news/best-hospitals/articles/2009/10/20/which-best-hospitals-are-best-and-worst-at-pain-management. Accessed December 1, 2011.

57. Coley KC, Williams BA, DaPos SV, Chen C, Smith RB. Retrospective evaluation of unanticipated admissions and readmissions after same day surgery and associated costs. *J Clin Anesth*. 2002;14(5):349-353.

58. Eckstrand JA, Habib AS, Williamson A, et al. Computerized surveillance of opioid-related adverse drug events in perioperative care: a cross-sectional study. *Patient Saf Surg*. 2009;3(1):18.

2

Challenges in the Management of Postsurgical Pain

Why Are We Not Doing a Better Job?

by Raymond S. Sinatra, MD, PhD

Introduction

Surgical caregivers and hospital administrators have expressed both surprise and dismay that despite the introduction of new analgesics and novel analgesic delivery systems, postsurgical pain remains suboptimally controlled.[1,2] Many ask why are we not doing a better job? A number of factors appear to be responsible for inadequate pain management, including:

- Lack of sufficient physician training
- Misconceptions and inappropriate patient expectations
- Intolerable analgesic adverse effects that contribute to noncompliance with prescribed therapy
- Analgesic gaps.[3]

Other factors, including underprescription as well as overprescription of opioid analgesics, not planning or allowing time for wound-site infiltration or regional blockade, misconceptions regarding use of NSAIDs, and overreliance on anesthesiologists and other caregivers to provide analgesic therapy, have been implicated as reasons why surgeon-directed management of postsurgical pain often remains suboptimal (**Table 2.1**).[3,4]

TABLE 2.1 — Factors Responsible for Lack of Improvement in Postsurgical Pain Management

• Educational deficits (uninformed, misinformed caregivers)
• Patient misinformation (unrealistic expectations, overconcern regarding addiction risks)
• Lack of "pain service" supervision (dedicated anesthesiology, surgical-, or nurse-directed protocol development and 24-hour coverage)
• Analgesic gaps (pain developing in a PACU, following transition in therapy and following hospital discharge)
• Technology failures (IV infiltration, pump misprogramming, epidural, or nerve block catheter dislodgement)
• Opioid "monotherapy" (overreliance on IV and oral opioids)
• Opioid dependency (not recognizing or adjusting therapy for opioid-tolerant and hyperalgesic patients)

Educational Deficits and Their Impact on Optimal Pain Management

Physician misconceptions regarding analgesic therapy are often the result of educational deficits and misinformation gained during medical training. Medical school and postgraduate training programs have historically placed a low educational emphasis on pain management.[5] Deficiencies in appreciating pain physiology and pathophysiology, plus a lack of didactic and bedside training in assessment, therapeutic options, and analgesic dosing, have contributed to the mindset in which postsurgical pain is often considered a low-priority clinical-management issue. While surgeons do not want their patients to unduly suffer, they may express indifference to aggressive interventional pain management, rationalizing that pain is a normal response to surgical injury and its intensity will progressively diminish during the healing process.[5]

Common educational deficits include:

- Nonrecognition of pain-related pathophysiologic responses and their impact on perioperative morbidity, particularly in elderly, obese, and high-risk populations[6]

- Negative attitudes towards opioids and exaggerated addiction concerns, resulting in a reluctance to prescribe them[7]
- Negative attitudes regarding NSAIDs, neural blockade with local anesthetic, duration of action of infiltrated local anesthetics and other multimodal analgesic options, resulting in the overprescription of opioids.

A classic example of misinformation and confusion regarding pain management involves the surgeon who requests that a highly effective epidural or continuous peripheral nerve block be discontinued because "after all, the patient has no pain." Other examples include surgeons who refuse to order preincisional neural blockade or perform wound-site infiltration because "it is not necessary," when in reality, they are concerned that it will delay the start time or duration of a case. Another common example involves highly risk-adverse caregivers who refuse to prescribe even a single dose of an IV NSAID or COX-2 inhibitor because of fears that they could negatively affect wound healing or bone remodeling.[8,9]

Surgeons can educate and positively influence patient expectations, thereby preparing them to better cope with postsurgical pain. Patients receiving realistic, unbiased pain management education prior to total hip arthroplasty were found to be significantly less anxious just before surgery than uninformed patients. They experienced less pain following surgery and were able to stand sooner.[10] Unfortunately, many surgeons, in an effort to allay presurgical anxiety, provide no information or deliberate misinformation. Those who inform patients that they will be using a pain pump or will be getting a nerve block and will not have any pain are actually doing a disservice, as patients will still have considerable pain and may become very dissatisfied with the effectiveness and quality of therapy. Studies have shown that in most settings, patients will report pain intensity scores of 3 to 5 with optimal IV-PCA opioid administration, and no nerve block can be guaranteed to be 100% effective.[11]

Underprescription of Opioid Analgesics

Although opioids are generally considered the foundation of analgesic therapy and treatment of choice for moderate to severe postsurgical pain, a relatively low proportion of patients actually receive prescriptions adequate to control their discomfort.[12,13] There is evidence to suggest that some surgeons withhold opioids because of:

- Confusion regarding addiction
- Regulation of controlled substances
- An exaggerated fear of legal liability and regulatory scrutiny.

A high proportion of physicians expressed fear of addiction as a reason against the use of opioid analgesics—approximately 28% believed that patients receiving opioids for pain relief were at significant risk for addiction, and an even greater proportion of physicians (39%) were concerned about addiction if a family member were to be prescribed morphine.[7] The fact that nurses commonly underadminister physician-prescribed doses may further compound the problem of analgesic undermedication.

A study by Orgill and associates[14] showed that surgeons underadministered opioids to inpatients with moderate to severe pain following total laryngectomy. To make matters worse, patients actually received significantly lower doses than that prescribed by their surgeons, and remarkably, no patient received the recommended minimum daily dose of morphine for adequate management of moderate-severe pain. Additionally, a relatively large number of patients (35%) continued to experience pain due to inadequate analgesic therapy yet only 22% had their opioid dose increased.

Patient concerns about the abuse and addiction potential of opioid analgesics are another barrier to appropriate use of these agents. A survey of 250 postsurgical patients revealed that of those who would choose a nonopioid agent for pain management (72%), almost half made their choice based on fear of addiction.[15] In contrast to the negative attitudes expressed by physicians and patients towards opioid therapy, studies have shown that when opioid analgesics are administered under proper physician supervision, treatment is associated with very low rates of opioid misuse. The apparent discrepancy between perceptions about the abuse potential of opioids and the actual risk of abuse supports the urgent need for improved physician and patient education with respect to the appropriate use of opioid analgesics for pain management.

Overreliance on Opioid Monotherapy

In contrast to those who underprescribe opioids, a growing number of surgeons rely almost exclusively on this class of analgesics for acute pain management, and many prescribe relatively large doses despite fears of respiratory depression and other adverse events and the potential for diversion and abuse. In a recent study looking at common inpatient surgical procedures in a large database of surgical patients, >95% of patients received opioids either on or after their surgical procedure.[16] Many of these caregivers prescribe opioids as monotherapy and feel comfortable with dosing regimens that employ small doses for mild to moderate pain, administration of more opioids for moderate-to-severe pain, and even more opioids for severe-to-very–severe pain (**Figure 2.1**).

While opioid uptitration appears to be rational, these monotherapeutic dosing protocols generally fail as patients suffer increasing adverse events and intolerability in relation to increasing exposure and elevations

FIGURE 2.1 — Postsurgical Opioid Analgesic Monotherapy

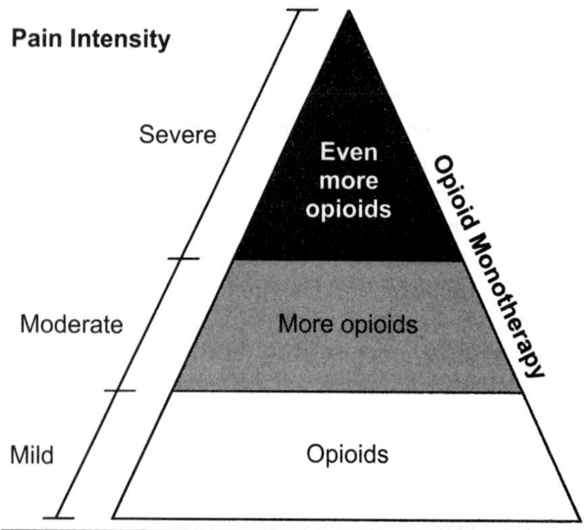

Opioid monotherapy suggests that postsurgical pain can be controlled by increasing opioid dose in proportion to the patient's pain-intensity complaint. The flaw in this dosing strategy is that increasing opioid dose results in increasing intolerability. This limits opioid dose and the effectiveness of pain management.

in CNS levels of drug. The overall effectiveness of any form of analgesic therapy consists of a balance between efficacy and overall tolerability. Opioids by themselves may not provide a useful balance in acute pain settings. High opioid-dose exposure or opioid "burden" is the key factor responsible for annoying side effects and occurs in a large proportion of patients prescribed IV or oral opioids.[15,17] Symptoms may become so intolerable that they negatively influence the success of analgesic therapy. Many patients refrain from prescribed dosing and choose to suffer moderate-to-severe discomfort rather than experience dose-associated adverse events. These patients suffer in silence rather than alerting the surgical office or risk "offending" their surgeons with complaints related to analgesic choice and dosing regimen.

In recent years, opioid-dose intolerance has become one of the most significant and widespread causes of poorly controlled acute pain.[17,18] In a systematic review that analyzed postsurgical opioid-associated adverse effects from multiple controlled observational trials, 31% of patients reported an adverse GI event, most commonly nausea, vomiting, ileus, or constipation.[18] Sedation and somnolence were the most commonly reported CNS effects (30.3%) (**Figure 2.2**). Other common adverse events included itching (18.3%), urinary retention (17.5%), and respiratory events (2.8%).

Oderda and coworkers[19] evaluated opioid-related adverse drug events (ADEs) in 60,722 postsurgical patients; 2.7% of patients experienced an ADE and the most common side effects were nausea and vomiting (67%) and pruritus (33.5%). Patients experiencing an opioid ADE had statistically significant increases in

FIGURE 2.2 — Opioid-Related Adverse Events Commonly Observed in Postsurgical Patients

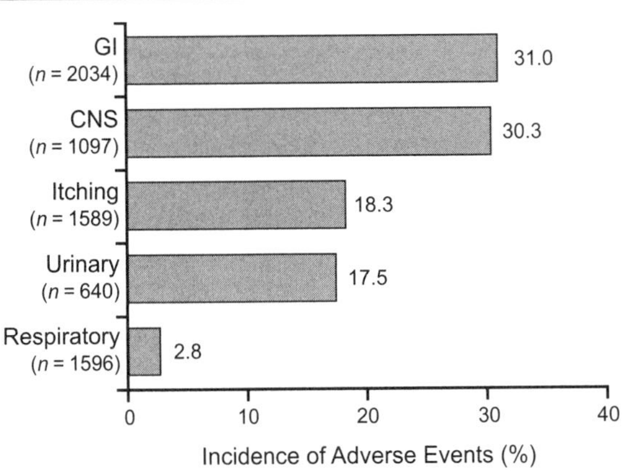

Data from a review of 45 randomized controlled trials

Wheeler M, et al. *J Pain*. 2002;3(3):159-180.

length of hospital stay (0.53 days) and increased hospital cost (16%), which averaged $840. Retrospective matched-cohort trials have found that elderly patients and those treated with higher doses of opioids are more likely to experience an ADE than those receiving lower doses (**Figure 2.3**).[20,21] In a similar study presented in 2011, Oderda and colleagues showed this difference to be nearly twice as much as their original study (increase in LOS of 1.1 days and increased hospital costs of $1614). Advanced age increased the risk factor for opioid-related ADEs and their impact on increased LOS and hospital costs. Importantly, the incidence of opioid-related ADEs in this national data set was 19.4% and if an opioid-related ADE occurred, the chance of becoming an LOS outlier increases by 214% and the chance of becoming a total cost outlier increases by 36% compared with patients who did not experience an opioid-related ADE (**Figure 2.4**).[16]

FIGURE 2.3 — Postsurgical Opioid-Related Nausea and Vomiting Appear to Be Dose Dependent

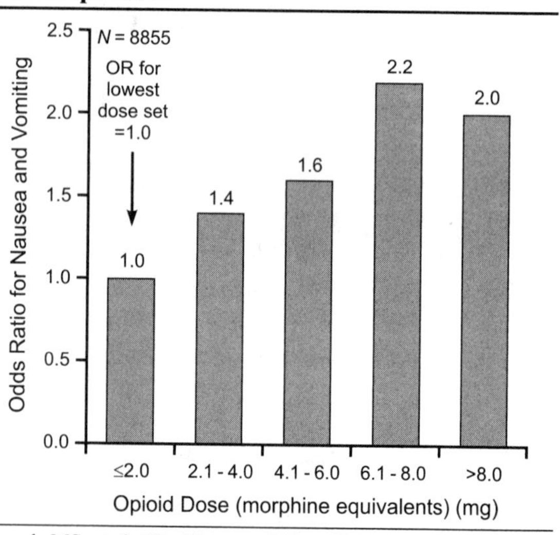

Cepeda MS, et al. *Clin Pharmacol Ther*. 2003;74(2):102-112.

FIGURE 2.4 — National Postsurgical Opioid Outlier Study

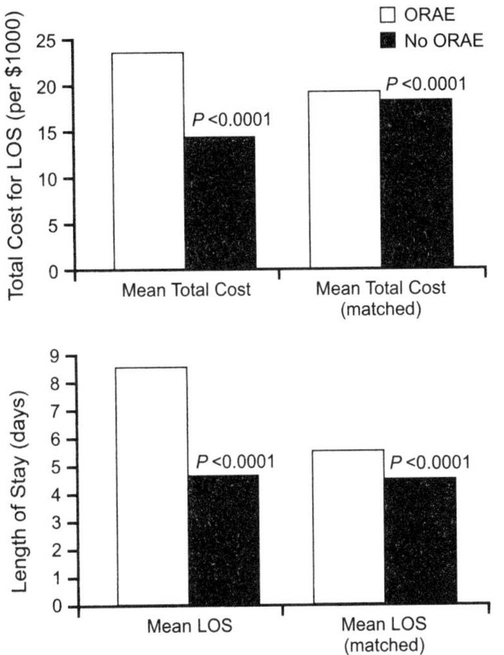

This recent study identified relationships between opioid-related adverse events (ORAEs) and increased length of hospital stay (LOS)/total cost in patients at least 18 years of age between September 2008 and August 2010. Individuals with an ORAE (n=45,342) were matched to those without an ORAE (n=135,941). Incidence of ORAEs was 19%. ORAEs increased mean LOS of 5.2 days (SD 3.5) vs 4.1 days (SD 2.8) (P<0.0001). ORAEs increased mean total cost of hospitalization $18,309 (SD 11,267) vs $17,281 (SD 10,209) ($P$<0.0001). The expected increased cost of a single ORAE utilizing adjusted cost variation modeling from baseline cost was $1614.

Oderda GM, et al. Poster presented at: 46th ASHP Midyear Clinical Meeting and Exhibition; December 4-8, 2011; New Orleans, LA. Poster 3-185.

One factor that increases risks for opioid intolerance and potential toxicity is the fact that surgeons often prescribe opioids according to standardized protocols despite marked patient variability in age, weight, and drug tolerance/dependency. This "one dose size fits all" dosing philosophy can lead to overdose and intolerance in frail elderly patients or subtherapeutic dosing in vigorous adults. Therapy should always be individualized for age-related differences in drug clearance and elimination, as well as effects on the CNS.

A common example of overstandardization is seen with IV-PCA morphine or hydromorphone order sets. Surgical orders often specify the same loading dose, bolus dose, lockout interval, and 4-hour limits for 30-year-old and 70-year-old patients and for less invasive vs highly invasive procedures. In recent years, an increasing number surgical procedures are being performed in patients with chronic opioid dependencies. Postsurgical IV-PCA orders for these patients are rarely adjusted or increased to compensate for opioid tolerance and, again, the same bolus dose given to a naïve individual is prescribed to a patient taking oxycodone 100 mg daily for chronic pain.[22]

As mentioned earlier, dose-dependent opioid adverse effects often prevent dosing to maximal efficacy and can be a contributing factor to patients' discontinuation of therapy. Many patients may choose to cope with pain rather than continue to experience intolerable opioid side effects.[15,17] This attitude was observed in preoperative and postsurgical interviews of 50 patients undergoing abdominal surgery, in which patients were asked to choose from among several hypothetical treatments with different characteristics reflecting the balance between analgesia and side effects. Overall, the severity of side effects was considered a more important consideration for therapy than the degree of pain relief, suggesting that many patients were willing to "trade" analgesic efficacy for a reduction in side effect severity (**Figure 2.5**).[17]

FIGURE 2.5 — Avoidance of GI Side Effects Is the Foremost Concern of Surgical Patients

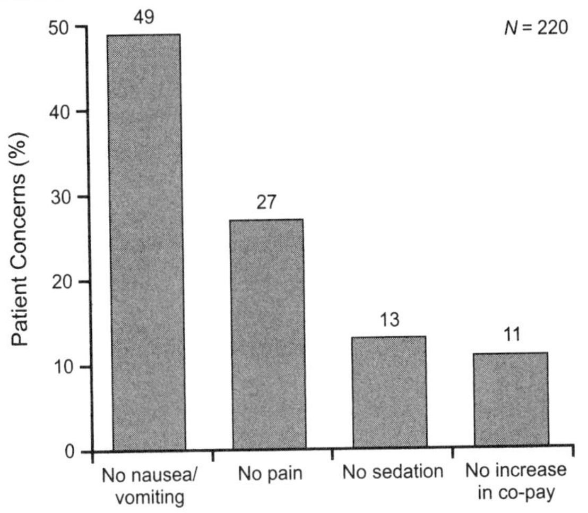

In a relative ranking of patient concerns, avoiding postoperative nausea and vomiting was the most important in this study.

Eberhart LH, et al. *Br J Anaesth*. 2002;89(5):760-761.

Thus many surgeons and patients alike share a difficult dilemma in that prescription of subtherapeutic opioid doses are often well tolerated yet provides inadequate pain relief, while prescription of higher, more effective doses often elicits an increased incidence of adverse events and suboptimal pain relief if dosing is discontinued. The answer may reside in the use of analgesic regimens to reduce the opioid burden and improve tolerability while still maintaining analgesic efficacy.

Analgesic Gaps

Analgesic gaps are specific time periods during postsurgical recovery when pain is unrelieved. These gaps may explain in part why the overall effectiveness of postsurgical pain management has not improved over the last 15 years.[3,4,23] For example, a patient may be extremely comfortable for many hours following major surgery, then a sudden change in analgesic delivery or change in patient activity may lead to dramatic increases in pain intensity. When patients are surveyed prior to hospital discharge, they remember these short, yet highly uncomfortable intervals, and rank overall pain relief and satisfaction lower than it could have been if the "gap" had not occurred. Common causes of analgesic gaps include (**Table 2.2**):

- Technology failures
- Pain following transition from an interventional technique to oral analgesics
- Pain following hospital discharge.

TABLE 2.2 — Analgesic Gaps: Specific Time Periods When Pain Is Unrelieved

- Pain in PACU (intraop analgesic deficiency or lack of local anesthetic wound infiltration)
- Pain during transport to and from procedures
- Technology failures (IV infiltration, pump misprogramming, catheter dislodgement)
- Transition from regional, neuraxial, or IV-PCA
- Inadequate analgesic prescriptions for home discharge

Patients experiencing severe pain in the PACU are the result of "anesthetic gaps" in which opioids or neural blockade is either withheld or administered in subtherapeutic doses. It may take many minutes to hours of opioid loading by PACU nurses to overcome this analgesic deficiency, which patients recall all too vividly.

Analgesic delivery systems that are complex, invasive, or involve multiple steps for analgesic administration have more frequent system-related events (SREs) or problems that must be addressed by health care providers. For IV-PCA opioids, infiltration of the IV line is a frequently reported SRE that results in an ineffective subcutaneous (SC) deposition of drug and increasing pain and discomfort. In this regard, the average patient may need to have their IV restarted 2.3 times just to maintain a site for PCA. A survey showed that there can be as many as 125 steps and six to eight different healthcare personnel involved in setting up and maintaining PCA therapy. This represents significant potential for error, including incorrect programming and device malfunctions and overdosing or underdosing errors.[24-27] The use of opioids and potential misprogramming of opioid pumps carry a considerable risk to the patient. From January 1995 to 2003, the Joint Commission found that 21% of medication error-related sentinel events involved opioids, and of those, 98% resulted in a fatal occurrence.[27] Two percent of opioid medication errors result in patient harm. If a PCA pump is involved, the chance for patient harm increases 3.5-fold.[27]

Another contributing factor for analgesic gaps is the disparity or inequity in the quality of health care based on age, gender, ethnicity, or race. It is well documented that although the overall health of Americans has improved over the past few decades, those improvements are not shared equally among all racial groups, particularly in the management of pain in both emergency room and postsurgical settings.[27-29] Elderly or disorientated patients may do poorly with PCA and should probably be offered alternative forms of analgesic delivery. It is not uncommon to find these patients attached to the PCA device yet complaining of severe pain as they have no idea how to locate or when to activate the button, or mistake it for a call button.[24]

Technology failures with epidural and peripheral nerve catheters are also responsible for analgesic gaps. The success rate of epidural catheters is about 70%, which means that the inherent potential failure of epidural technology is about 30%.[30] A common situation is pain related to catheter dislodgement following turning, physical therapy, or ambulation. Epidural solutions are very dilute in terms of local anesthetic and/or opioid dose and rapidly become subtherapeutic if the catheter is no longer in the epidural space. Epidural and peripheral nerve infusion–related medication errors can also occur, particularly if there is a kink in the catheter line, insufficient solution left in the medication bag, or the device becomes unplugged and the batteries lose their charge. Finally, since any infusion pump requires caregiver input, there is the potential that someone is going to use the wrong solution and infusion settings.[23,24] The surgeon and nursing staff should contact anesthesiology caregivers immediately to evaluate any interventional technique that is not providing effective pain relief. Adjustments in catheter position and bolusing of drugs generally reestablishes analgesia, although in some situations, catheters may need to be replaced or an alternative analgesic technique provided.

Inappropriate management of the transition between interventional infusion techniques and oral medications also contributes to analgesic gaps. Continuous epidural or peripheral infusions with local anesthetics, the use of single-dose longer-acting local anesthetics and IV-PCA can provide excellent pain control but often such therapy is discontinued and replaced by a surgical order for as-needed opioids, which provide suboptimal analgesia.[31] While many surgeons have moved away from short-acting opioids as primary postsurgical analgesics and employ NSAIDs or acetaminophen, many continue to prescribe hydrocodone or oxycodone preparations that provide only 3 or 4 hours of pain relief. This creates a cycle in which the patient has to request or take pain medication frequently and experiences periods of inadequate analgesia over and over again. Since acute surgical pain has a constant component with periods of exacerbation, caregivers are increasingly prescribing sustained-release morphine or oxycodone as a continuous approach to pain management.[32]

REFERENCES

2

1. Warfield CA, Kahn CH. Acute pain management. Programs in U.S. hospitals and experiences and attitudes among U.S. adults. *Anesthesiology*. 1995;83(5):1090-1094.
2. Apfelbaum JL, Chen C, Mehta SS, Gan TJ. Postoperative pain experience: results from a national survey suggest postoperative pain continues to be undermanaged. *Anesth Analg*. 2003;97(2):534-540.
3. Carr DB, Reines HD, Schaffer J, Polomano RC, Lande S. The impact of technology on the analgesic gap and quality of acute pain management. *Reg Anesth Pain Med*. 2005;30(3):286-291.
4. Ng A, Hall F, Atkinson A, Kong K, Hahn A. Bridging the analgesic gap. *Acute Pain*. 2000;3(4):1-6.
5. Wilder-Smith OH, Möhrle JJ, Martin NC. Acute pain management after surgery or in the emergency room in Switzerland: a comparative survey of Swiss anaesthesiologists and surgeons. *Eur J Pain*. 2002;6(3):189-201.
6. Vanderah TW. Pathophysiology of pain. *Med Clin North Am*. 2007;91(1):1-12.
7. Weissman DE, Joranson DE, Hopwood MB. Wisconsin physicians' knowledge and attitudes about opioid analgesic regulations. *Wis Med J*. 1991;90(12):671-675.
8. Adolphson P, Abbaszadegan H, Jonsson U, Dalén N, Sjöberg HE, Kalén S. No effects of piroxicam on osteopenia and recovery after Colles' fracture. A randomized, double-blind, placebo-controlled, prospective trial. *Arch Orthop Trauma Surg*. 1993;112(3):127-130.
9. Wheeler P, Batt ME. Do non-steroidal anti-inflammatory drugs adversely affect stress fracture healing? A short review. *Br J Sports Med*. 2005;39(2):65-69.
10. Giraudet-Le Quintrec JS, Coste J, Vastel L, et al. Positive effect of patient education for hip surgery: a randomized trial. *Clin Orthop Relat Res*. 2003;(414):112-120.
11. Borgeat A, Schäppi B, Biasca N, Gerber C. Patient-controlled analgesia after major shoulder surgery: patient-controlled interscalene analgesia versus patient-controlled analgesia. *Anesthesiology*. 1997;87(6):1343-1347.
12. Rupp T, Delaney KA. Inadequate analgesia in emergency medicine. *Ann Emerg Med*. 2004;43(4):494-503.

13. McNamara RM, Rousseau E, Sanders AB. Geriatric emergency medicine: a survey of practicing emergency physicians. *Ann Emerg Med.* 1992;21(7):796-801.

14. Orgill R, Krempl GA, Medina JE. Acute pain management following laryngectomy. *Arch Otolaryngol Head Neck Surg.* 2002;128(7):829-832.

15. Gan TJ, Lubarsky DA, Flood EM, et al. Patient preferences for acute pain treatment. *Br J Anaesth.* 2004;92(5):681-688.

16. Oderda GM, Gan TJ, Robinson SB, Johnson B. Opioid-related adverse events increase length of stay and drive up total cost of care in a national database of postsurgical patients. Poster presented at: 46th ASHP Midyear Clinical Meeting and Exhibition; December 4-8, 2011; New Orleans, LA. Poster 3-185.

17. Eberhart LH, Morin AM, Wulf H, Geldner G. Patient preferences for immediate postoperative recovery. *Br J Anaesth.* 2002;89(5):760-761.

18. Wheeler M, Oderda GM, Ashburn MA, Lipman AG. Adverse events associated with postoperative opioid analgesia: a systematic review. *J Pain.* 2002;3(3):159-180.

19. Oderda GM, Evans RS, Lloyd J, et al. Cost of opioid-related adverse drug events in surgical patients. *J Pain Symptom Manage.* 2003;25:276-283.

20. Oderda GM, Said Q, Evans RS, et al. Opioid-related adverse drug events in surgical hospitalizations: impact on costs and length of stay. *Ann Pharmacother.* 2007;41(3):400-406.

21. Cepeda MS, Farrar JT, Baumgarten M, Boston R, Carr DB, Strom BL. Side effects of opioids during short-term administration: effect of age, gender, and race. *Clin Pharmacol Ther.* 2003;74(2):102-112.

22. Mitra S, Sinatra RS. Perioperative management of acute pain in the opioid-dependent patient. *Anesthesiology.* 2004;101(1):212-227.

23. Hankin CS, Zhang M. Analysis of reported adverse events associated with intravenous patient-controlled analgesia: findings from the FDA Center for Devices and Radiological Health manufacturer and user facility device experience (MAUDE) database. Poster presented at: 2005 Summer Meeting of the American Society of Health-System Pharmacists; June 11-15, 2005; Boston, MA.

24. Viscusi ER, Schechter LN. Patient-controlled analgesia: finding a balance between cost and comfort. *Am J Health Syst Pharm.* 2006;63(8 suppl 1):S3-13.

25. USP Center for the Advancement of Patient Safety. *USP Quality Review: Patient-Controlled Analgesia Pumps*. Rockville, MD: USP Center for the Advancement of Patient Safety; 2004. The United States Pharmacopeial Convention, Inc. publication PSF053DM.

26. Cohen MR, Smetzer J. Patient-controlled analgesia safety issues. *J Pain Palliat Care Pharmacother*. 2005;19(1):45-50.

27. Sikirica V, Hicks RW, Nelson WW, Schein J, Cousins D. Frequency, type, and cause of patient-controlled analgesia (PCA) vs non-PCA medication errors in the USP MEDMARX database. Paper presented at: 41st ASHP Midyear Clinical Meeting; December 3-7, 2006; Anaheim, CA.

28. Green CR, Anderson KO, Baker TA, et al. The unequal burden of pain: confronting racial and ethnic disparities in pain. *Pain Med*. 2003;4(3):277-294.

29. Atherton MJ, Feeg VD, el-Adham AF. Race, ethnicity, and insurance as determinants of epidural use: analysis of a national sample survey. *Nurs Econ*. 2004;22(1):6-13.

30. Agency for Healthcare Research and Quality, US Department of Health and Human Services. *AHRQ Focus on Research: Disparities in Health Care*. Rockville, MD: Agency for Healthcare Research and Quality, 2002. AHRQ Pub. No. 02-M027.

31. Ready LB. Acute pain: lessons learned from 25,000 patients. *Reg Anesth Pain Med*. 1999;24(6):499-505.

32. Chen PP, Chui PT, Ma M, Gin T. A prospective survey of patients after cessation of patient-controlled analgesia. *Anesth Analg*. 2001;92(1):224-227.

3 Pain Definitions and Assessment

How Pain is Defined

By Raymond S. Sinatra, MD, PhD

3

Introduction

Pain has been defined as the conscious awareness of tissue injury yet several other definitions have also been proposed. The IASP suggests that pain is "an unpleasant sensory and emotional experience associated with actual or potential tissue damage."[1,2] McCaffery and Beebe defined pain as "whatever the experiencing person says it is, existing whenever the experiencing person says it does" unless proven otherwise by poor adherence to an agreed treatment plan.[3]

Pain is a complex physiologic process that can be classified in terms of its[1,4]:

- Intensity (mild, moderate, severe)
- Duration (acute, convalescent, chronic)
- Mechanism (physiologic, nociceptive, inflammatory, neuropathic)
- Clinical context (postsurgical, malignancy-related, myelopathic, degenerative).

Pain detection or nociception follows the activation of specialized transducers called nociceptors, which are the peripheral endings of A-delta (Aδ) and c-type sensory fibers. Pain perception follows afferent transmission of noxious impulses to higher cortical centers where it is localized, characterized, and graded in intensity (**Figure 3.1**).

FIGURE 3.1 — Pain Processing Involves Detection, Transmission, and Perception

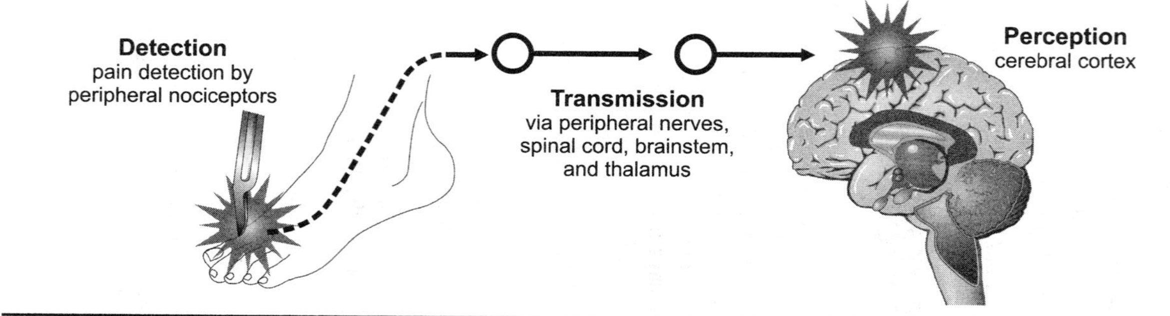

Pain Processing Theory

A number of theories have been proposed to explain pain processing and perception.[4-6] The earliest attempt to describe pain processing was the "specificity theory of nociception" proposed by Descartes. The specificity theory suggested that different nerve fiber types specifically discriminated between different forms of noxious and non-noxious sensations. Sydenham later proposed the "intensity theory of nociception," suggesting that the intensity of the peripheral stimulus determined the type of sensation perceived. The "gate-control theory" proposed by Melzack and Wall[5] suggested that nerve fibers of differing size and specificity stimulated second-order spinal neurons termed transmission (T) cells. Depending upon the degree of facilitation or inhibition, T cells fire at varying intensities and send noxious information to the brain. Large non-noxious sensory fibers also activate inhibitory "SG cells" that "close the processing gate" by suppressing T cells. Descending inhibition from higher CNS centers can also close the gate (**Figure 3.2**). While portions of the gate-control theory have been disproved, the idea of pain "gating" in the spinal cord remains valid.

The most recent proposal to describe pain processing is termed the "sensitization theory of nociception."[6] Following tissue injury, inflammatory mediators and cytokines sensitize peripheral nociceptors, resulting in exaggerated responses to painful and nonpainful stimuli. Noxious impulses in turn sensitize second-order transmission neurons in the dorsal horn, resulting in central sensitization. Central sensitization results in secondary hyperalgesia and spread of the hyperalgesic area to nearby uninjured tissues. Inhibitory interneurons and descending inhibitory fibers modulate and suppress spinal sensitization, while analgesic undermedication and poorly controlled pain favors sensitization (see *Chapter 5*).

FIGURE 3.2 — The Gate-Control Theory of Pain Processing and Perception

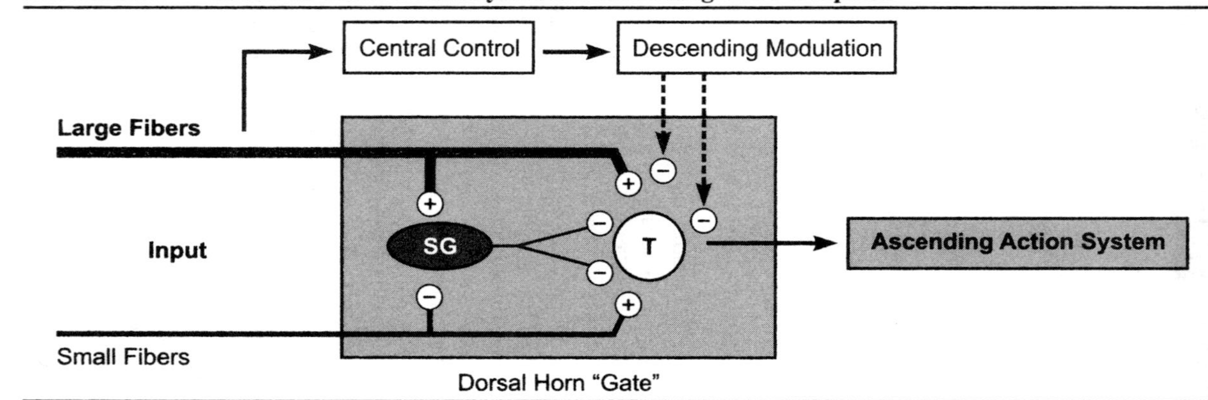

Key: SG, substantia gelatinosa cell; T, second-order transmission.

Modified from Melzack R, Wall PD. *Science*. 1965;150(699):971-979.

Pain Definitions

Several forms of pain have been defined[4,7,8]:

- Physiologic pain
- Nociceptive pain
- Neuropathic pain.

3

Physiologic Pain

Physiologic pain is brief, rapidly perceived, nontraumatic discomfort that identifies a potentially dangerous stimulus. This adaptive alerting response involves cortical perception and localization, as well as reflex withdrawal that prevents and/or minimizes tissue injury. Physiologic pain is also associated with learned avoidance and adaptation that can modify future behavior. We learn quickly to never again touch a hot flame.

Nociceptive Pain

Nociceptive pain results from the activation of physiologically normal nerve fibers in response to tissue injury.[4] This is the primary mechanism for acute pain produced in the postsurgical setting. In addition to cellular damage and neural irritation, humoral mediators and peripheral inflammatory responses play major roles in its initiation and progression. Nociceptive pain can be further divided into the following subtypes:

- Somatic pain
- Visceral pain.

Somatic pain is well-localized, sharp, crushing, or tearing pain that follows traumatic injury to dermatomally innervated structures. It includes cutaneous, muscular, and ligamentous pain, but also includes headache and osteogenic pain. In contrast, visceral nociceptive pain is poorly localized, nondermatomal specific discomfort that is usually described as dull, cramping, or colicky.

Visceral pain includes discomfort related to bowel obstruction, first-stage labor, dilation of hollow viscus, early appendicitis, and peritoneal irritation. Visceral pain is mediated by free nerve endings in GI organs and peritoneum that respond to irritation or distention. Referred pain is a special form of visceral pain that radiates in a somatic dermatomal pattern.[7,8]

■ Neuropathic Pain

Neuropathic pain results from irritation, infection, degeneration, transection, or compression injury to nervous tissue. It is usually characterized as burning, electrical, and/or shooting in nature. Pain following injury to sensory nerves is termed causalgia or chronic regional pain syndrome II. Pain associated with injury or abnormal activity of sympathetic fibers is termed reflex sympathetic dystrophy or chronic regional pain syndrome I. Neuropathic pain is often associated with peripheral and central sensitization, secondary hyperalgesia, and alterations in sympathetic tone and regional perfusion.[4,7,8]

A common characteristic of neuropathic pain is the coexistence of neurologic deficits and sensory abnormalities in the setting of increased pain sensation. These abnormalities include:

- Hyperpathia, or increased or exaggerated pain intensity with minor stimulation
- Allodynia, in which non-noxious sensory stimulation is perceived as painful
- Dysesthesia/paresthesia, which are unpleasant sensations at rest or following touch and movement.[8-10]

Differences between physiologic, nociceptive, and neuropathic pain are described in the **Table 3.1**.

Pain Temporality and Duration

■ Acute Pain

Acute pain is an adaptive physiologic response that follows traumatic injuries and surgery. It has two primary components[1]:

- Sensory discriminative component
- Affective-motivational component.

TABLE 3.1 — Pain Categories and Symptoms

Category	Cause	Symptom	Examples
Physiologic	Brief exposure to a noxious stimulus	Rapid, yet brief pain perception	Touching a pin or hot object
Nociceptive/ inflammatory	Somatic or visceral tissue injury with mediators affecting intact nervous tissue	Moderate-to-severe pain, described as crushing or stabbing; usually worsens after the first 24 hours	Surgical pain, traumatic pain, sickle-cell crisis
Neuropathic	Damage or dysfunction of peripheral nerves or CNS	Burning or electrical shock-like pain	Neuropathy, nerve transection, postherpetic neuralgia
Mixed	Combined somatic and nervous-tissue injury	Combinations of symptoms; soft tissue pain plus radicular pain	Low-back pain, back surgical pain, amputation

The *sensory discriminative component* describes the location and quality of the stimulus. It is characterized by rapid response, short latency to peak response, and short duration of action. Noxious information is conveyed by rapidly conducting Aδ fibers and monosynaptic transmission to the sensory cortex. This component rapidly identifies the site of injury or potential injury and initiates reflexive/cognitive withdrawal responses.[2]

The *affective-motivational component* underlies the suffering and emotional components of pain and is responsible for learned avoidance and other adaptative and nonadaptative behavioral responses. The affective motivational component is mediated by slowly conducting C fibers and polysynaptic transmission to the limbic cortex. It is responsible for continued pain perception, suffering, pain-related behaviors, hyperalgesia, and reflex spasm (splinting behavior). It is also responsible for immobilization and protection of the injury site.

Hyperalgesia describes a state of increased pain sensitivity and enhanced perception following acute injury, which is related to peripheral release of intracellular or humoral noxious mediators[9,10] (see *Chapter 5*). Primary hyperalgesia or peripheral sensitization describes an altered state of sensibility in which the intensity of painful sensation induced by noxious stimulation at the site of injury is greatly increased. Secondary hyperalgesia or central sensitization describes increased pain sensation at sites adjacent to the injury site and associated reflex muscle spasm.[8-10]

In general, acute pain is limited in duration (1 to 14 days) and is associated with temporal reductions in intensity (**Figure 3.3**). Optimally controlled acute pain may be mild to moderate at rest but generally worsens during movement (effort-dependent or incident pain). Poorly controlled acute pain is associated with peripheral sensitization, spinal facilitation, hypothalamic/adrenal responses, and emotional/behavioral changes.[11]

FIGURE 3.3 — Temporal Differences in Postsurgical Pain

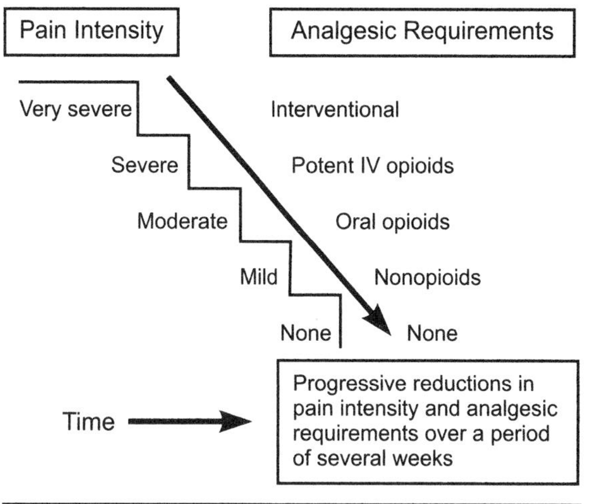

■ Rehabilitative/Convalescent Pain

A subacute pain state associated with convalescence and rehabilitation may persist for 1 to 2 months after surgery or traumatic injury. Paticnts may experience moderate to severe incident pain and require opioid analgesics for sleep and mobilization. Severe rehabilitative pain has a negative impact on physical therapy, return to normal functionality, and quality of life.

■ Chronic Pain

Chronic pain refers to persistent or progressively increasing discomfort beyond the normal time frame of healing. An alternative definition is moderate-to-severe discomfort persisting ≥3 months following tissue injury (postsurgical pain syndrome) or initial symptoms of cellular degeneration (osteoarthritic disease). The etiologic classification of chronic pain refers to the clinical context in which pain perception takes place and can be categorized as benign, malignancy-related, postsurgical, neuropathic, degenerative, or mixed.[4,12]

Chronic pain is often associated with sensitization and plasticity changes in the peripheral and CNS that facilitate pain transmission and impair intrinsic noxious modulatory mechanisms. Transition from acute pain to chronic pain involves ongoing peripheral and central sensitization, persistent hyperalgesia, the development of neuropathic symptoms, and maladaptive emotional responses (pain behavior)[6,9,10] (**Figure 3.4**). Patients with chronic pain may be troubled by a persistent pain state that remains constant or gradually increases in frequency and intensity (malignancy-associated pain, osteoarthritis) or an intermittent pain state that has peaks (flare) and troughs in intensity (vasculopathic pain, gout, low back pain). Others may present with a combination of persistent pain plus intermittent flare and complaints of pain that is constant or gradually increasing, with episodes of increased intensity or flare (rheumatoid arthritis, neuropathic pain).

Chronic pain may also be characterized by its localization. Peripheral pain is associated with ongoing nociceptor sensitization, neuropathic injury, and stimulation of sympathetic efferents. Myelopathic pain is associated with spinal injuries and includes localized irritative and compression-related pain, radicular pain, and skeletal muscular irritability. Central pain describes pain syndromes that follow CNS injury (poststroke, CNS tumor) that are generally ill defined/poorly localized and difficult to treat.

While some forms of chronic pain have an unclear etiology and unpredictable course, most begin as acute inflammatory or neuropathic pain. An increasing body of evidence suggests that severe acute pain, analgesic undermedication, nerve injury, and genetic variabilities are responsible for the development of chronic pain.[13,14]

Although acute and chronic pain have distinguishing characteristics, there is often overlap, making the diagnosis and management of pain challenging. Differences between acute and chronic pain are outlined in **Table 3.2**.

FIGURE 3.4 — Transitions From Acute to Persistent Pain

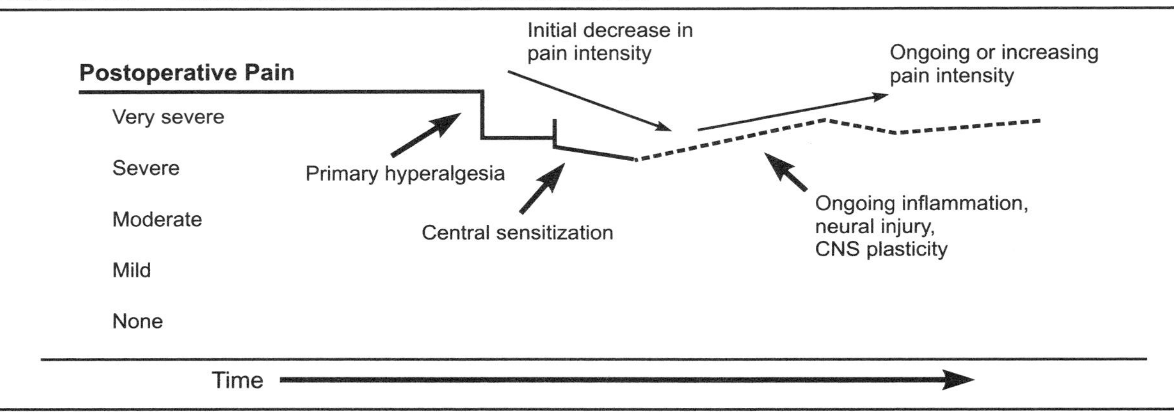

3

TABLE 3.2 — Differences Between Acute and Chronic Pain

Characteristics	Acute Pain	Chronic Pain
Cause	Usually obvious tissue damage	Multiple causes (malignancy, benign)
Onset	Distinct onset	Gradual or distinct onset
Duration	Short, well-characterized duration	Persists after 3 to 6 months of healing
Resolution	Resolves with healing	Can be a symptom or diagnosis
Biological function	Serves a protective function	Serves no adaptive purpose
Treatment	Effective therapy is available	May be refractory to treatment

Qualitative Aspects of Pain Perception

Appreciating the clinical features of the different types of pain not only helps properly classify pain and its etiology but also helps to guide the often complex multimodal medical management that accompanies pain management. The health care provider must be detailed in attaining the qualitative factors and history associated with a patient's pain. Qualitative aspects of pain perception are outlined in **Table 3.3**.

Finally, it is well-recognized that certain acute traumatic and chronic pain conditions are associated with a mixture of nociceptive inflammatory and neuropathic pain. For example, tissue injury and a marked inflammatory response following laparotomy or thoracotomy initiates a somatic nociceptive component responsible for incisional and muscular pain, while peritoneal or pleuritic irritation is responsible for a visceral nociceptive component. Neural injury related to retraction or transection initiates a neuropathic component. Clinical pain complaint, intensity of symptoms, pain characteristics, and choice of analgesic are related to the extent of inflammation, visceral vs somatic nociception, and neural tissue injuries.

TABLE 3.3 — Pain Characteristics: Based on Focused Physical Examination and History

Temporal
- Onset
- Duration
- Periodicity

Variability
- Constant
- Effort dependent
- Waxing and waning
- Episodic "flare"

Intensity
- Average pain
- Worst pain
- Least pain
- Pain with activity of living

Topography
- Focal
- Dermatomal
- Diffuse
- Referred
- Superficial
- Deep

Character
- Sharp
- Aching
- Cramping
- Stabbing
- Burning
- Shooting

Exacerbating/Relieving
- Is pain worse at rest, with movement, or no difference?

Quality of Life
- Does pain interfere with movement, ambulation, daily life tasks, or work?

REFERENCES

1. Bonica JJ. Definitions and taxonomy of pain. In: Bonica JJ, ed. *Management of Pain*. 2nd ed. Philadelphia, PA: Lea & Febiger; 1990.
2. Pain terms: a list with definitions and notes on usage. Recommended by the IASP Subcommittee on Taxonomy. *Pain*. 1979;6(3):249.
3. McCaffery M, Beebe A. *Pain: Clinical Manual for Nursing Practice*. St. Louis, MO: CV Mosby; 1989.
4. Raj PP. Taxonomy and classification of pain. In: Kreitler S, Beltrutti D, Lamberto A, Niv D. *The Handbook of Chronic Pain*. Hauppauge, NY: Nova Biomedical Books; 2007.
5. Melzack R, Wall PD. Pain mechanisms: a new theory. *Science*. 1965;150(699):971-979.
6. Woolf CJ, Salter MW. Neuronal plasticity: increasing the gain in pain. *Science*. 2000;288(5472):1765-1769.
7. Bonica JJ. Anatomic and physiologic basis of nociception and pain. In: Bonica JJ, ed. *Management of Pain*. 2nd ed. Philadelphia, PA: Lea & Febiger; 1990: 28-94.
8. Fields HL, Martin JB. Pain: pathophysiology and management. In: Braunwald E, Fauci AS, Kasper DL, Hauser SL, Longo DL, Jameson JL, eds. *Harrison's Principles of Internal Medicine*. 15th ed. New York, NY: McGraw-Hill; 2001.
9. Mannion RJ, Woolf CJ. Pain mechanisms and management: a central perspective. *Clin J Pain*. 2000;16(suppl 3):S144-S156.
10. LaMotte RH, Thalhammer JG, Robinson CJ. Peripheral neural correlates of magnitude of cutaneous pain and hyperalgesia: a comparison of neural events in monkey with sensory judgments in human. *J Neurophysiol*. 1983;50(1):1-26.
11. Sinatra RS, Bigham M. The anatomy and pathophysiology of acute pain. In: Grass JA, ed. *Problems in Anesthesiology*. Philadelphia, PA: Lippincott-Raven; 1997.
12. Agency for Health Care Policy Research. *Management of Cancer Pain. Clinical Practice Guidelines No. 9*. Rockville, MD: US Department of Health and Human Services; 1994. AHCPR Publication No. 94-0592.
13. Perkins FM, Kehlet H. Chronic pain as an outcome of surgery. A review of predictive factors. *Anesthesiology*. 2000; 93(4):1123-1133.
14. Kehlet H, Jensen TS, Woolf CJ. Persistent postsurgical pain: risk factors and prevention. *Lancet*. 2006;367(9522):1618-1625.

4 Surgical Pain Pathways

by Raymond S. Sinatra, MD, PhD

Introduction

Analgesics mediate their effects by targeting receptors or inhibiting the release of noxious substances in:

- Peripheral tissues
- Sensory nerves
- Spinal cord
- Brain.

Understanding the anatomic pathways and key neurochemical mediators involved in noxious detection and perception is key to optimizing the management of acute and chronic pain.[1,2]

The following steps underlie pain perception:

1. Peripheral noxious mediators that result from surgical procedures activate nociceptor endings via a process termed "transduction."
2. Noxious impulses are delivered to the spinal cord dorsal horn via afferent "conduction."
3. "Transmission" refers to synaptic transfer of noxious impulses from primary afferents to second-order cells in the dorsal horn.
4. "Modulation" describes inhibition of noxious transmission within the dorsal horn. Modulation includes local enkephalinergic interneuron inhibition.

   "Facilitation" refers to activation of *N*-methyl-D-aspartate acid (NMDA) receptors located on second-order cells in the dorsal horn. Neuronal activation is associated with a "windup" or increase in firing frequency and exaggerated responses to non-noxious and noxious input.

"Spinal reaction" includes reflex activation of sympathetic and motor efferent fibers, increases in vascular and skeletal muscle tone, and associated hypertension, tachycardia, and muscle spasm/splinting.

5. "Descending inhibition" refers to the suppression of pain transmission by descending contacts from noradrenergic and enkephalinergic cells in the brainstem, midbrain, and cerebral cortex.
6. Cortical "perception" includes neocortical sites of pain identification and localization as well as limbic centers responsible for emotional and suffering components of pain.
7. "Supraspinal reaction" describes cortical responses, including fear, anxiety, depression, and other pain-related behaviors, as well as pituitary-hypothalamic responses including the release of stress hormones, and neuropeptides (**Figure 4.1**).

Peripheral Pain Processing

Pain processing begins with the activation of peripheral nociceptors. These unmyelinated endings of sensory nerve fibers are found in skin, bone, muscle, peritoneal linings, and every organ in the body except the brain.[1,3] Nociceptors act as peripheral pain detectors that respond to a variety of noxious thermal, pressure-related, and chemical insults. Cellular damage following surgical dissection or trauma leads to the release of intracellular hydrogen and potassium ions that directly activate nociceptors. Arachidonic acid, a component of damaged cell membranes, is also released. Arachidonic acid is rapidly converted by COX-2 into prostaglandins (PGE_2, and later PGH_2).[4] COX-2 is also upregulated at the site of injury. Prostaglandins are highly inflammatory substances that also function as primary nociceptor activators. They exacerbate tissue swelling and pain at the site of

FIGURE 4.1 — Steps Involved in Pain Detection, Transmission, Perception, and Reaction

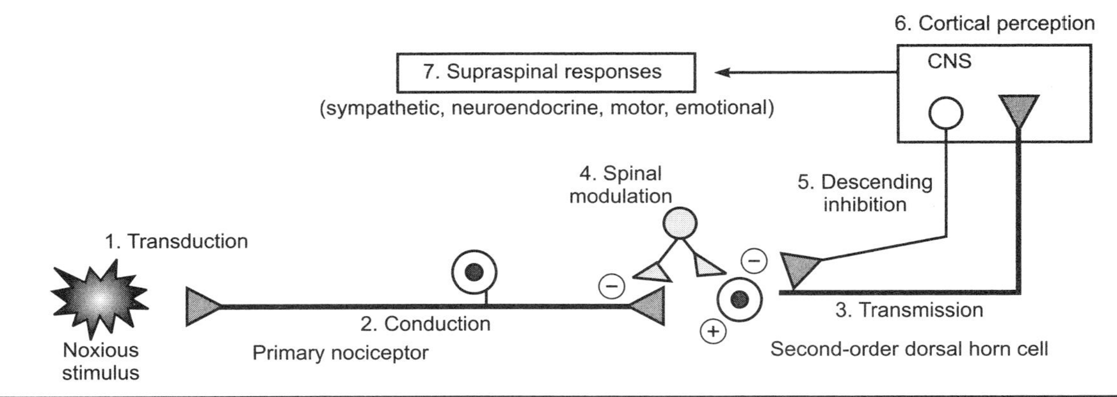

injury and play a role in the development of primary hyperalgesia and secondary hyperalgesia.[4,5] COX-2 is also upregulated in spinal cord and brain, where PGE_2 appears to play a role in central sensitization and plasticity changes that underlie the development of chronic pain[5,6] (**Figure 4.2**). This locally induced inflammatory state provides the rationale for the current local infiltration of NSAIDs into surgical wounds, as well as the rationale for the development of extended-duration NSAID preparations (ie, DepoNSAID). Other noxious mediators, including bradykinin, leukotrienes, histamine, calcitonin gene-related peptide (CGRP), and substance P, maintain a state of irritability and ongoing depolarization of nociceptors.[1] Bradykinin is a markedly algesic substance that has direct activating effects on peripheral nociceptors. Substance P is a neuropeptide released from the unmyelinated afferent fibers. The proinflammatory effects of substance P include:

- Vasodilation and plasma extravasation
- Degranulation of mast cells
- Chemoattraction and proliferation of leukocytes
- Cytokine release.

Histamine is stored in mast-cell granules and is released by substance P and other noxious mediators. The effects of histamine are mediated by its interaction with specific receptors, resulting in vasodilation and edema and swelling resulting from the enhanced permeability of postcapillary venules. Serotonin or 5-hydroxytryptamine (5-HT) is stored in the dense-body granules of platelets. 5-HT enhances microvascular permeability.[2,7]

Specialized ion channels termed "transient receptor potential voltage-one" (TRPV-1) depolarize nociceptor endings and initiate action potentials in sensory nerve axons. The TRPV-1/capsaicin ion channel has been well described. It contains a central ion channel that permits inward Ca^{++} and Na^{+} currents following stimulation by H^{+} ions, heat, and direct application of

FIGURE 4.2 — Peripheral and Central Effects of Prostaglandins and Their Role in Acute and Chronic Pain

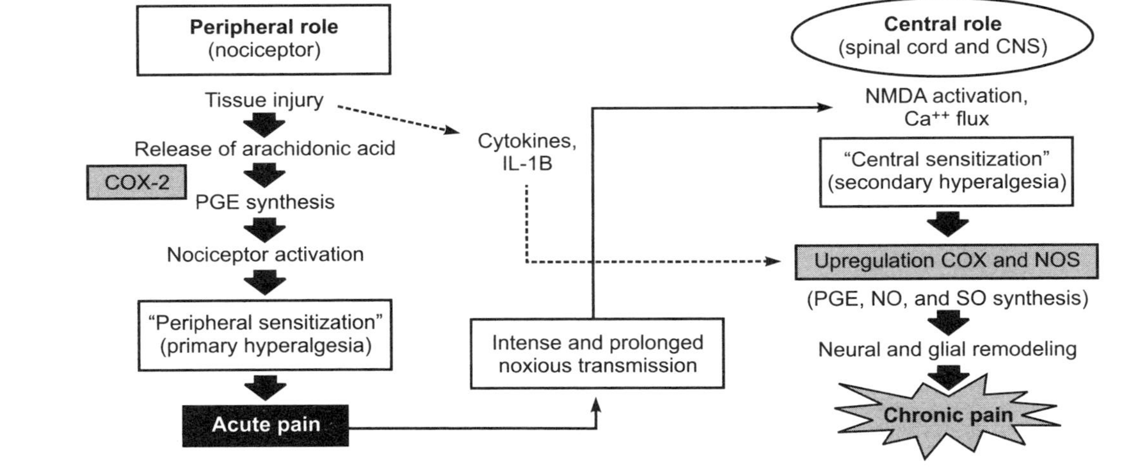

capsaicin, the active chemical compound found in hot pepper. The inward flux of Ca^{++} via TRP ion channels is responsible for generator potentials that summate and depolarize the distal axonal segment. Thereafter a sodium-mediated action potential conducts noxious signals centrally to terminals in dorsal horn. The "noxious soup" of local, humoral, and neural mediators released following acute tissue injury, as well as the nociceptor response to peripheral injury, are summarized in **Figure 4.3**.

Primary noxious conducting nerves are either unmyelinated C fibers or larger, myelinated Aδ fibers that innervate a wide variety of tissues.[1] Aδ fibers transmit "first pain," a rapid (within 1 second) well-localized, discriminative sensation (sharp, stinging) of short duration. Perception of first pain alerts the individual of actual or potential tissue injury and initiates reflex withdrawal mechanisms. Smaller, unmyelinated C fibers (termed polymodal nociceptive fibers) respond to mechanical, thermal, and chemical injuries. C fibers mediate the sensation of "second pain," which has a delayed latency (seconds to minutes) and is perceived as a diffuse burning or stabbing sensation that persists for a prolonged period of time.[2]

Spinal Cord

Aδ and C fibers enter the spinal cord dorsal horn and terminate predominantly in laminae II (substantia gelatinosa) and V. Their terminal endings make synaptic contact with second-order dorsal horn neurons and in response to noxious stimulation, release excitatory amino acids (EAAs) or peptide-based neurotransmitters[8,9] (**Figure 4.4**). EAAs, glutamate, and aspartate mediate rapid short-duration depolarization of dorsal-horn neurons. Peptides, substance P, and neurokinin are responsible for delayed and long-lasting depolarization. EAAs activate AMPA receptors, resulting in an influx of Na^+ ions and cellular depolarization. This allows noxious signals to be rapidly transmitted to supraspinal sites of perception.

In the setting of continued high-frequency noxious stimulation, activated AMPA receptors initiate voltage-mediated priming of NMDA receptors.[2,8,9] The NMDA receptor is a 4-subunit membrane protein that regulates inflow of Na^+ and Ca^{++} and cellular outflow of K^+. Priming, in turn, dislodges a magnesium ion "plug" that normally blocks the NMDA ion channel. Following dislodgement of Mg^{++}, a rapid influx of Ca^{++} ions occurs. Accumulation of intracellular Ca^{++} initiates a series of neurochemical and neurophysiologic changes that influence acute pain processing. Second-order spinal neurons become highly sensitized and fire rapidly and independently of further sensory stimulation.[8-11] This process is termed "windup." Local anesthetic blockade prior to injury can prevent windup but cannot reverse windup once it is well established.[8,11] Woolf and others have shown that NMDA activation, windup, and central sensitization are responsible for central sensitization and secondary hyperalgesia.[8,11]

Intracellular Ca^{++} ions also activate inducible enzymes, including nitric oxide synthase (NOS) and COX-2. Peptides, such as sP and CGRP, are responsible for delayed and long-lasting depolarization of second-order dorsal horn neurons. Substance P binding at neurokinin-1 (NK-1) receptors synergistically activates NMDA receptors.[9,10] Following activation of NK-1, second messengers, cyclic adenosine monophosphate (cAMP) and phosphokinase-A (PKA), are synthesized and mediate a number of cellular changes, including slow priming of NMDA receptors, second messenger cascades, and genome activation. Synthesis of acute-phase proteins together with increased intracellular and extracellular PGE and nitric oxide (NO) are responsible for transcription dependent neural plasticity changes that facilitate pain transmission. **Figure 4.5** provides an overview of noxious excitation and its effect on second-order dorsal horn neurons.

FIGURE 4.3 — The "Noxious Soup" of Pain Detection

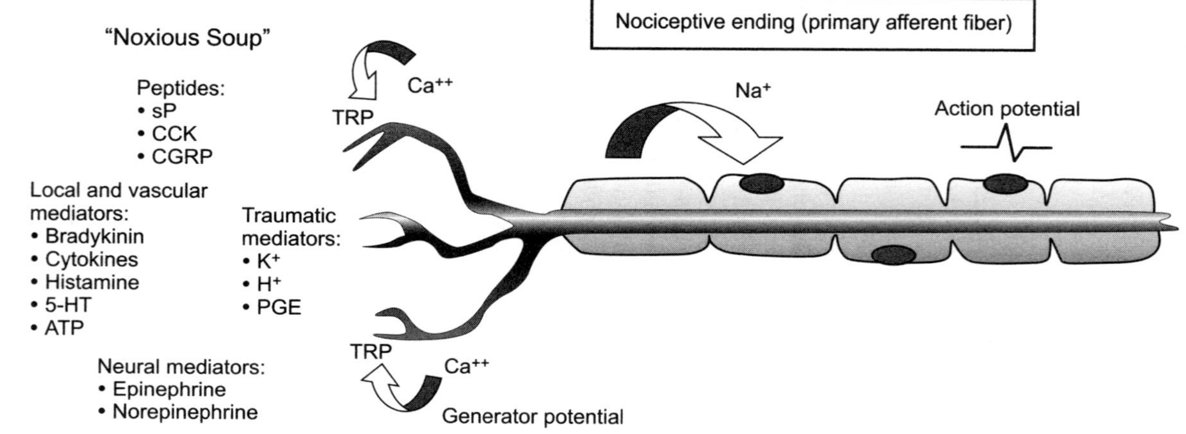

Key: 5HT, serotonin; ATP, adenosine triphosphate; Ca++, calcium ion; CCK, cholecystokinin; CGRP, calcitonin gene-related peptide; H+, hydrogen ion; K+, potassium ion; Na+, sodium ion; PGE, prostaglandin; TRP, tubular reabsorption of phosphate.

Pain is detected by unmyelinated nerve endings, termed nociceptors, that innervate skin, bone, muscle, and visceral tissues. Nociceptor activation initiates a depolarizing Ca^{++} current or generator potential. Generator potentials depolarize the distal axonal segment and initiate an inward Na^{+} current and self-propagating action potential. Following tissue injury, cellular mediators (potassium, hydrogen ions, and prostaglandin released from damaged cells, as well as bradykinin released from damaged vessels) activate the terminal endings (nociceptors) of sensory afferent fibers. Prostaglandin, synthesized by COX-2, is responsible for nociceptor sensitization and plays a key role in peripheral inflammation. The release of these mediators and others, such as serotonin (5-HT) and cytokines, creates a "noxious soup" that exacerbates the inflammatory response, recruits adjacent nociceptors, and results in primary hyperalgesia. Reflex sympathetic efferent responses may further sensitize nociceptors directly by releasing noradrenaline and indirectly by stimulating further release of bradykinin and sP, leading to peripheral vasoconstriction and trophic changes.

Sinatra R. 2007.

4

FIGURE 4.4 — Pain Pathways and Synaptic Contacts Within the Spinal Cord

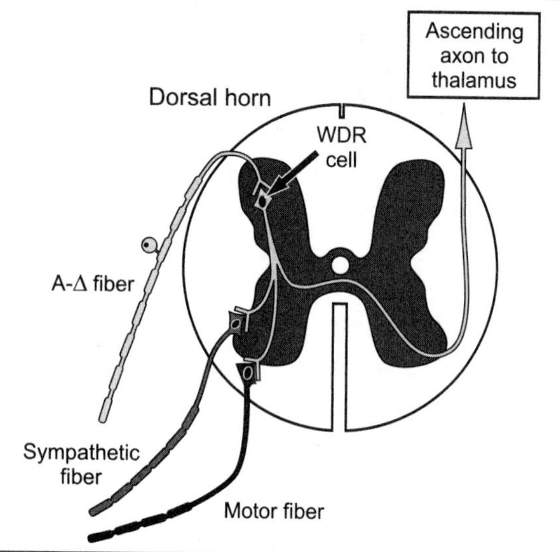

Afferent noxious fibers enter and synapse with second-order NS or WDR cells in the dorsal horn. Projections from second-order cells contact efferent motor and sympathetic cell bodies in the spinal cord and also ascend to supraspinal sites.

Second-order dorsal horn neurons are of two main types:

- Nociceptive-specific neurons (NS), which respond exclusively to noxious impulses from C fibers
- Wide-dynamic range neurons (WDR), which respond to both noxious and innocuous stimuli.[3]

Low-frequency C fiber stimulation results in nonpainful sensory transmission, while higher-frequency stimulation leads to gradual increases in WDR neuronal discharge. Dorsal horn inhibitory neurons and descending inhibitory axons release enkephalin (EK), norepinephrine (NE), and other modulatory substances that decrease the excitability of WDR cells. Thus, the magnitude of noxious stimulation, balanced by the activity of inhibitory cells, can influence sensory processing in WDR neurons, resulting in transmission of either noxious or innocuous messages to the thalamus. Studies by Woolf and others[8-10] showed that prolonged high-frequency stimulation leads to NMDA receptor activation and a sustained burst of WDR activity termed windup. Windup results in central sensitization and secondary hyperalgesia. In certain settings, central sensitization may then lead to neurochemical/neuroanatomic changes (plasticity) and the development of chronic pain.[8-10]

Modulation

The concept of modulation refers to pain suppressive mechanisms within the spinal cord dorsal horn and at higher levels of the brainstem and midbrain. In the spinal cord, this intrinsic "breaking mechanism" inhibits pain transmission at the first synapse between the primary noxious afferent and second-order WDR and NS cells, thereby reducing spinothalamic relay of noxious impulses. Spinal modulation is mediated by the inhibitory actions of endogenous analgesic compounds, released from spinal interneurons and terminal endings of inhibitory axons that descend from central grey locus ceruleus and other supraspinal sites.[2,3] Endogenous analgesics including ENK, NE, and γ-aminobutyric acid (GABA) activate opioid, α-adrenergic, and other receptors that either inhibit release of glutamate (Glu) from primary nociceptive afferents or diminish postsynaptic responses of second-order NS or WDR neurons. The balance between excitatory mediators and the inhibitory effects of endogenous analgesics adjusts K^+ ion flux and the firing frequency of dorsal horn cells. Endogenous opioids, including the ENKs and endorphin, modulate pain transmission by activating pre- and postsynaptic μ, κ, and δ receptor subtypes. μ-opioid receptors are primarily responsible for mediating spinal and supra-

FIGURE 4.5 — Targets of Excitatory Noxious Mediators on Second-Order Cells

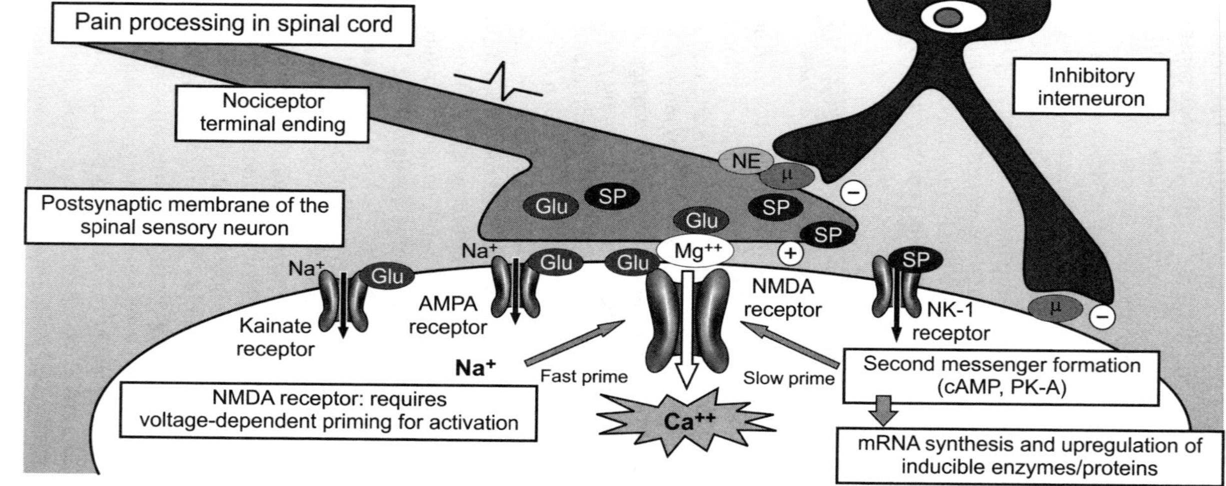

Key: AMPA, α-amino3-hydroxy-5-methylisoxazole-4-proprionic acid; Ca^{++}, calcium ion; cAMP, cyclic adenosine monophosphate; Glu, glutamate; Mg^{++}, magnesium ion; mRNA, messenger ribonucleic acid; Na^{+}, sodium ion; NE, norepinephrine; NK-1, neurokinin 1; NMDA, N-methyl-D-aspartate; PK-A, protein kinase A; SP, substance P.

Glutamate is the primary excitatory agonist for noxious transmission. Glutamate activates specific binding sites located on AMPA, kainate, and NMDA receptors. Ion channels on activated AMPA and kainate receptors allow Na^{+} to enter and depolarize the cell. Changes in intracellular voltage rapidly prime the NMDA receptor and allow a Mg^{++} plug to be dislodged. Following dislodgement, an inward flux of Ca^{++} is initiated. Glutamate binding to NMDA receptors maintains the inward Ca^{++} flux. Substance P binds and activates NK-1 receptors. This receptor upregulates second messengers, including cAMP and PK-A, which slowly prime and maintain excitability of NMDA receptors. Activation of second messengers in turn upregulates inducible enzymes, initiates transcription of mRNA, and mediates synthesis of acute reaction proteins. These changes increase neuronal excitability and underlie subsequent plasticity.

4

spinal analgesia, euphoria, and respiratory depression. κ subtypes mediate spinal analgesia, as well as sedative/hypnotic effects of opioids. Opioid binding at μ receptors activates coupled G-proteins (Gi/o), which in turn inhibit the neuronal cAMP pathway. Adenylate cyclase is suppressed, and production of cAMP and PKA is markedly reduced. Reductions in cAMP and inhibition of K^+ influx decrease neuronal excitability.[1,2]

The modulatory effects of NE are mediated by activation of postsynaptic α-adrenergic receptors. The ability of α-adrenergic receptors to suppress noxious transmission in the spinal cord is nearly equivalent to that observed following binding and activation of opioid receptors and forms the basis of tricyclic antidepressant–mediated analgesia.

Primary and Secondary Hyperalgesia

Hyperalgesia defines a state of increased sensitivity and enhanced pain perception following acute injuries such as incisional, crush, amputation, and blunt trauma. Clinically, patients experience pain in response to stimuli that normally would not be perceived as painful[12-14] (**Figure 4.6**). The hyperalgesic region may extend dermatomes above and below the area of injury and is associated with ipsilateral and occasionally contralateral muscular spasm/immobility. Primary hyperalgesia describes an altered state of sensibility (allodynia, hyperpathia) in which the intensity of painful sensation induced by noxious and non-noxious stimulation is greatly increased (**Table 4.1**). Primary hyperalgesia is related to peripheral release of intracellular or humoral noxious mediators.[12] It is responsible for increases in dynamic or "effort-dependent" pain, in which discomfort during ambulation, coughing, and physical therapy is significantly increased. Continued activation of nociceptors secondary to neural compression, stretch, infection, hematoma, and edema can result in prolonged disability and impaired rehabilitation. Secondary hyperalgesia reflects the

FIGURE 4.6 — Stimulus-Response Alterations Observed With Hyperalgesia

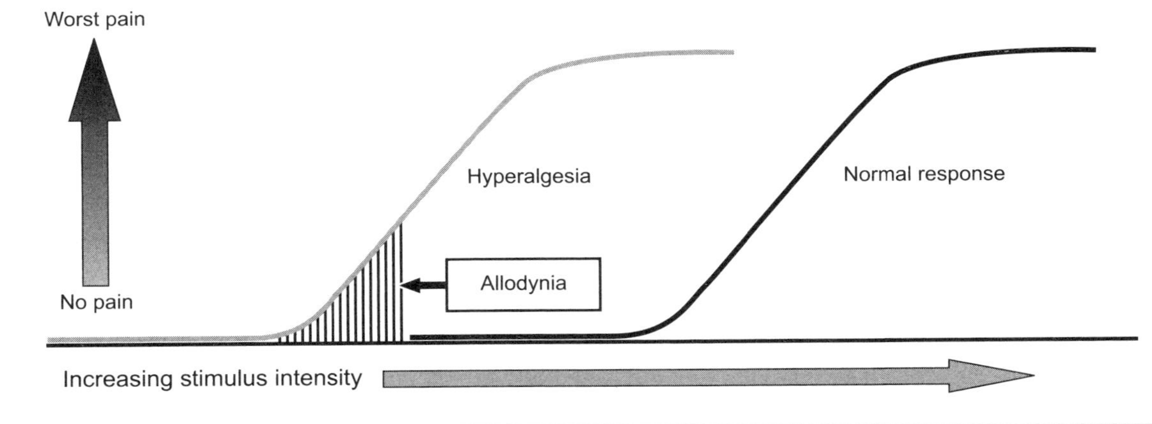

TABLE 4.1 — Abnormal Sensations Associated With Hyperalgesia

Hyperpathia
• Increased or exaggerated pain intensity with minor stimulation
Allodynia
• Non-noxious sensory stimulation is perceived as painful
Dysesthesia
• Unpleasant sensation at rest or movement

activation and sensitization of spinal cord neurons and associated reflex responses.[13,14] Ongoing barrages of noxious impulses transmitted via high-threshold afferents overwhelm tonic inhibitory mechanisms and trigger long-lasting changes in dorsal horn neurons. Following sensitization, WDR and NS cells become increasingly responsive to innocuous peripheral stimuli over widened dermatomal receptive fields.[14] This has important clinical implications since pain sensation usually requires more intense stimulation. As a result, effort-dependent pain is more intense, rehabilitation may be compromised, and the risk of persistent pain increases.[15,16]

Ascending Pathways

Ascending pain pathways transmit nociceptive impulses to the thalamus and cerebral cortex, where pain sensation is perceived, characterized, and responded to. Axons from NS and WDR dorsal horn cells may either synapse with sympathetic anterolateral horn cells, anterior horn motor neurons, or project to brainstem, midbrain, and thalamus[3,15] (**Figure 4.7**). Several ascending spinal tracts are involved in the transmission of nociceptive information from the dorsal horn to supraspinal sites—the spinothalamic tract (STT) is considered the most important pathway. The STT is divided into two tracts: the lateral neo-spinothalamic tract (nSTT) and the more medial paleo-

FIGURE 4.7 — An Anatomical Overview of Pain Pathways

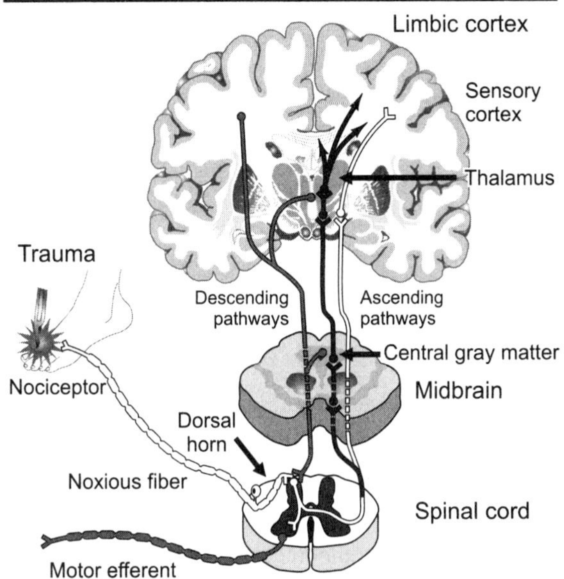

Noxious information is conveyed from peripheral nociceptors to the dorsal horn via unmeylinated and myelinated noxious fiber. Second-order spinal neurons send impulses rostrally via two distinct pathways: the neospinothalamic and paleospinothalamic tracts. These cells also activate motor and sympathetic efferents within the spinal cord. Ascending tracts make contacts in the brainstem and midbrain, central gray matter, and thalamus. Projections are then made with frontal and limbic cortex. Descending fibers emanating from cortex, hypothalamus, and brainstem project to the spinal cord to modulate pain transmission.

spinothalamic tract (pSTT). The nSTT projects directly to the neothalamus. The neothalamus is a highly somatotopically organized region with cells conveying nociceptive impulses directly to the somatosensory cortex for rapid perception (localization) and prompt withdrawal from the noxious stimulus.[3] The pSTT is a slow multisynaptic pathway that projects to the reticular activating system (RAS), periaqueductal gray (PAG), and medial thalamus.[17] The medial thalamus is not somatotopically organized, and its cells project to the frontal and limbic cortex. The pSTT is associated with prolonged acute pain and chronic pain and is responsible for diffuse, unpleasant discomfort and suffering long after an injury has occurred. Nociceptive impulses transmitted by the pSTT lead to persistent supraspinal responses affecting circulatory, respiratory, and endocrine function and underlie emotional and behavioral responses such as fear, anxiety, helplessness, and learned avoidance.[2,3]

Descending Control of Pain

Descending neural pathways inhibit pain perception and efferent responses to pain.[2,15,18] The cerebral cortex, hypothalamus, thalamus and brainstem centers PAG, nucleus raphes magnus (NRM), and locus caeruleus (LC) send descending axons to the brainstem and spinal cord that modulate pain transmission in the dorsal horn.[3,15,17] These axonal terminals either inhibit release of noxious neurotransmitters from primary afferents or diminish the response of second-order neurons to the noxious input. Several neurotransmitters play critical roles in modulating pain transmission, including the endogenous opioids (ENK, dynorphin), GABA, and NE. The PAG is an enkephalinergic brainstem nucleus responsible for both morphine and stimulation-produced analgesia. Descending axons from the PAG project to nuclei in the reticular formation of the medulla, including NRM, then descend to the dorsal horn where they synapse with and inhibit WDR and NS neurons. Axon terminals from NRM project to dorsal horn, where they release serotonin and NE. Axons descending from LC modulate nociceptive transmission in the dorsal horn primarily via release of NE and activation of postsynaptic α_2-adrenergic receptors. The role of NE in this pathway may explain the analgesic effects of tricyclic antidepressants. GABAergic and enkephalinergic interneurons in the dorsal horn also provide local suppression of pain transmission.[15]

Conclusion

Pain transmission and perception involve not only peripheral receptors and sensory pathways, but also synaptic contacts in the spinal cord and brainstem. An overview of pain pathways and pain perception is presented in **Figure 4.7**. Knowledge of pain pathways and pain processing helps guide the surgeon with decisions regarding optimal use of analgesics and neural blockade, as well as factors that increase the intensity of acute pain and lead to the development of persistent pain states. Modulatory processes within the dorsal horn can either inhibit or facilitate pain transmission and initiate reflexive motor and sympathetic responses. Recent information suggests central sensitization and plasticity changes not only increase the severity of acute pain but are causative factors underlying the transition to persistent pain. In addition to their peripheral effects, humoral inflammatory factors (PGE, cytokines, interleukins) also play a role in the activation and sensitization of central sites involved in pain processing. Although acute pain initiates protective withdrawal and immobilization reflexes that minimize further tissue injury, chronic pain is persistent, serves no adaptive benefit, and can lead to long-term disability.

REFERENCES

1. Sinatra RS, Bigham M. The anatomy and pathophysiology of acute pain. In: Grass JA, ed. *Problems in Anesthesiology*. Philadelphia, PA: Lippincott-Raven; 1997.
2. Vadivelu N, Whitney C, Sinatra RS. Pain pathways. In: Sinatra RS, Viscusi G, DeLeon-Cassasola O, Ginsberg B, eds. *Acute Pain Management*. London, England: Cambridge Press; 2009.
3. Bonica JJ. Anatomic and physiologic basis of nociception and pain. In: Bonica JJ, ed. *The Management of Pain*. 2nd ed. Philadelphia, PA: Lea & Febiger; 1990:28-94.

4. Vane JR, Botting RM. New insights into the mode of action of anti-inflammatory drugs. *Inflamm Res*. 1995;44(1):1-10.
5. Ito S, Okuda-Ashitaka E, Minami T. Central and peripheral roles of prostaglandins in pain and their interactions with novel neuropeptides nociceptin and nocistatin. *Neurosci Res*. 2001;41(4):299-332.
6. Funk CD. Prostaglandins and leukotrienes: advances in eicosanoid biology. *Science*. 2001;294(5548):1871-1875.
7. Mannion RJ, Costigan M, Decosterd I, et al. Neurotrophins: peripherally and centrally acting modulators of tactile stimulus-induced inflammatory pain hypersensitivity. *Proc Natl Acad Sci U S A*. 1999;96(16):9385-9390.
8. Woolf CJ, King AE. Subthreshold components of the cutaneous mechanoreceptive fields of dorsal horn neurons in the rat lumbar spinal cord. *J Neurophysiol*. 1989;62(4):907-916.
9. Chaplan SR, Malmberg AB, Yaksh TL. Efficacy of spinal NMDA receptor antagonism in formalin hyperalgesia and nerve injury evoked allodynia in the rat. *J Pharmacol Exp Ther*. 1997;280(2):829-838.
10. Ji RR, Woolf CJ. Neuronal plasticity and signal transduction in nociceptive neurons: implications for the initiation and maintenance of pathological pain. *Neurobiol Dis*. 2001;8(1):1-10.
11. Malinow R, Malenka RC. AMPA receptor trafficking and synaptic plasticity. *Annu Rev Neurosci*. 2002;25:103-126.
12. LaMotte RH, Thalhammer JG, Robinson CJ. Peripheral neural correlates of magnitude of cutaneous pain and hyperalgesia: a comparison of neural events in monkey with sensory judgments in human. *J Neurophysiol*. 1983;50(1):1-26.
13. Woolf CJ. An overview of the mechanisms of hyperalgesia. *Pulm Pharmacol*. 1995;8(4-5):161-167.
14. Woolf CJ, Salter MW. Neuronal plasticity: increasing the gain in pain. *Science*. 2000;288(5472):1765-1769.
15. Mannion RJ, Woolf CJ. Pain mechanisms and management: a central perspective. *Clin J Pain*. 2000;16(suppl 3):S144-S156.
16. Woolf CJ, Mannion RJ. Neuropathic pain: aetiology, symptoms, mechanisms, and management. *Lancet*. 1999;353(9168):1959-1964.
17. Keay KA, Clement CI, Owler B, Depaulis A, Bandler R. Convergence of deep somatic and visceral nociceptive information onto a discrete ventrolateral midbrain periaqueductal gray region. *Neuroscience*. 1994;61(4):727-732.
18. Kehlet H. Surgical stress: the role of pain and analgesia. *Br J Anaesth*. 1989;63(2):189-195.

5

Multimodal Analgesia in the Postsurgical Patient

A Stepwise Approach to Postsurgical Analgesic Therapy

by Raymond S. Sinatra, MD, PhD

5

Introduction

Overreliance on a single class of analgesic commonly results in:

- Intolerable adverse events (AEs)
- Limited efficacy
- Diminished patient satisfaction.

In an effort to minimize dose-dependent AEs and potential toxicity associated with analgesic monotherapy, a growing number of surgical- and anesthesiology-based caregivers advocate a stepwise, multidrug approach to pain management. Several medical societies, including the ASA and the American College of Orthopedic Surgery, recommend balanced or "multimodal" analgesia and seamless perioperative administration rather than opioid monotherapy (**Table 5.1**).[1-3]

As described in *Chapter 2*, opioids have various idiosyncratic or dose-limiting side effects that curtail their practical efficacy as well as expose patients to dangerous AEs.[4-7] In addition to life-threatening respiratory depression, opioids increase:

- The risk of constipation and ileus, which can result in significant discomfort and a longer hospital stay
- Nausea and vomiting, which can lead to wound dehiscence and delayed recovery[4-6]

TABLE 5.1 — American Society for Anesthesiology Postsurgical Pain Practice Guidelines

Perioperative Techniques for Pain Management

Guidelines

- The literature supports the:
  - Efficacy and safety of three techniques used by anesthesiologists for perioperative pain control:
    - Epidural or intrathecal opioid analgesia
    - PCA with systemic opioids
    - Regional analgesic techniques, including but not limited to intercostal blocks, plexus blocks, and local anesthetic infiltration of incisions.
  - Analgesic efficacy of peripheral nerve blocks, eg:
    - Intercostal
    - Ilioinguinal
    - Interpleural
    - Plexus
  - Postincisional infiltration with local anesthetics for postoperative analgesia
- The literature is equivocal regarding the analgesic benefits of preincisional infiltration

Recommendations

- Anesthesiologists who manage perioperative pain should utilize therapeutic options such as epidural or intrathecal opioids, systemic opioid PCA, and regional techniques, after thoughtfully considering the risks and benefits for the individual patient. These modalities should be used in preference to intramuscular opioids ordered "as needed"
- The therapy selected should reflect the individual anesthesiologist's expertise, as well as the capacity for safe application of the modality in each practice setting
- Special caution should be taken when continuous infusion modalities are used, as drug accumulation may contribute to adverse events

Continued

TABLE 5.1 — *Continued*

Multimodal Techniques for Pain Management

Guidelines

- The literature supports the administration of two analgesic agents that act by different mechanisms via a single route for providing superior analgesic efficacy with equivalent or reduced adverse effects. Examples include:
  - Epidural opioids administered in combination with epidural local anesthetics or clonidine
  - IV opioids in combination with ketorolac or ketamine
- Dose-dependent adverse effects reported with administration of a medication occur whether it is given alone or in combination with other medications. For example:
  - Opioids may cause nausea, vomiting, pruritus, or urinary retention
  - Local anesthetics may produce motor block
- When compared with oral opioids alone, the literature is insufficient to evaluate the postoperative analgesic effects of oral opioids combined with:
  - NSAIDs (eg, ibuprofen, ketorolac)
  - COXIBs (eg, celecoxib, rofecoxib, parecoxib)
  - Acetaminophen
- The Task Force believes that NSAID, COXIB, or acetaminophen administration has a dose-sparing effect for systemically administered opioids
- The literature suggests that two routes of administration, when compared with a single route, may be more effective in providing perioperative analgesia Examples include:
  - Epidural or intrathecal opioid analgesia combined with IV, IM, oral, transdermal, or subcutaneous analgesics vs epidural opioids alone
  - IV opioids combined with oral NSAIDs, COXIBs, or acetaminophen vs IV opioids
- The literature is insufficient to evaluate the efficacy of pharmacologic pain management combined with nonpharmacologic, alternative, or complementary pain management when compared with pharmacologic pain management alone

Continued

TABLE 5.1 — *Continued*

Multimodal Techniques for Pain Management *(continued)* **Recommendations** • Whenever possible, anesthesiologists should employ multimodal pain management therapy • Unless contraindicated, all patients should receive an around-the-clock regimen of NSAIDs, COXIBs, or acetaminophen; in addition, regional blockade with local anesthetics should be considered • Dosing regimens should be administered to optimize efficacy while minimizing the risk of adverse events • The choice of medication, dose, route of administration, and duration of therapy should be individualized • Sedative, analgesic, and local anesthetics are all important components of appropriate analgesic regimens for painful procedures

Adapted from American Society of Anesthesiologists Task Force on Acute Pain Management. *Anesthesiology*. 2004;100(6):1573-1581.

- Urinary retention and CNS disturbance that result in increased LOS and hospital cost[4]
- Pruritis that can lead to patient discomfort.[4]

Multimodal Analgesia

Multimodal analgesia is defined as the simultaneous use of different analgesic agents or forms of analgesic delivery that suppress pain transmission in the peripheral and CNS.[8-11] Multimodal analgesic regimens can be designed to:

- Inhibit the release of noxious mediators
- Block conduction in sensory nerves
- Suppress pain perception in the CNS.

The multimodal analgesic concept is not unlike current multitherapeutic management of a variety of disease states, including hypertension, asthma, diabetes, and infection. The evolved standard of care in these common conditions is to use smaller, nontoxic doses of several different agents to control the disease process as opposed to utilizing any single agent at such a high dosage that one encounters dose-limiting adverse events associated with any single agent. It is the basis of current standards of care, including the management of hypertension where multiple agents with different mechanisms of action are now recommended. Another example is asthma, where it would be inappropriate to only address bronchoconstriction with an inhaled β-blocker without also addressing the inflammatory component with an inhaled corticosteroid. The basis of a multimodal strategy in the control of acute pain is similar.

5

Administration of agents having different mechanisms of action can provide important clinical benefits, including additive or synergistic effects and enhanced analgesic efficacy.[8,9] Because of measurable gains in overall analgesic effect, dose requirements of each respective agent may be reduced significantly. As a result, dose-related AEs are diminished and overall safety is increased.[9-11]

The downside of multimodal dosing regimens is that by definition, they:

- Require that more medications be administered
- May be more expensive
- Require a broader provider knowledge base to achieve maximal efficacy while avoiding drug-drug interactions and toxicity
- May pose compliance challenges for elderly patients in outpatient settings (**Table 5.2**).

A number of clinical trials have found that multimodal therapy results in greater analgesic uniformity and patient satisfaction than that observed with opioids alone and facilitates mobilization and rehabilitation.[7,8,10,11] In a meta-analysis of 52 randomized, placebo-controlled trials of multimodal analgesia vs opioid monotherapy, Elia and colleagues[12] reported that multimodal analgesia with NSAIDs or acetaminophen resulted in a 15% to 55% decrease in opioid dosing. They also noted significant reductions in pain intensity

TABLE 5.2 — Multimodal or Balanced Analgesia

Advantages
• Reduction in pain-intensity scores • Reduction in opioid-dose requirements (opioid-sparing effect) • Reduction in opioid side effects • Improved patient satisfaction • Improvement in surgical outcome (?)
Disadvantages
• Requires knowledge of multiple drugs, their pharmacokinetics and pharmacodynamics • Every analgesic has its own unique adverse event profile • May increase drug-drug interactions • Requires skills in regional and neuraxial analgesia • Possible postdischarge patient confusion and compliance issues

Kehlet H, et al. *Anesth Analg*. 1993;77(5):1048-1056; Elia N, et al. *Anesthesiology*. 2005;103(6):1296-1304; Sinatra RS, et al. *Reg Anesth Pain Med*. 2006;31(2):134-142.

at 24 hours and a reduced incidence of nausea/vomiting (from 29% to 22%) and sedation (from 15.4% to 12.7%) when compared with opioid monotherapy.

Multimodal analgesia involves the use of:

- Local-acting agents
- Local anesthetic infiltration and perineural blockade
- Reduced doses of opioid analgesics.

A list of multimodal analgesics advocated for acute pain management is shown in **Table 5.3**.

In some cases, opioids can be omitted completely from postsurgical order sets. Perhaps the best way caregivers can appreciate multimodal analgesia is to understand where and how different classes of analgesics interact within the pain transmission pathway (**Figure 5.1**). The following noxious generating and transmitting targets provide the rationale for nonopioid analgesics and analgesic adjuvants.

■ Transduction

Noxious transmission begins following activation of peripheral nociceptors, a process termed "transduction." Agents that modulate pain signaling at peripheral nociceptors include local anesthetics, NSAIDs, and COX-2 inhibitors (coxibs).[13,14] By reducing PGE synthesis, NSAIDs decrease inflammatory hyperalgesia and nociceptor sensitization. NSAIDs decrease the recruitment of leukocytes and the production of inflammatory cytokines. Some NSAIDs penetrate the blood-brain barrier and provide additional analgesia by diminishing PGE synthesis in the spinal cord and brain.[15]

Currently, two injectable NSAIDs, ketorolac (Toradol) and ibuprofen (Caldolor), are available for use in the postsurgical period. Injectable ibuprofen can be used pre-, intra-, and postsurgically. Ketorolac is associated with greater risk of hemorrhage and is approved only for postsurgical administration.[16,17] NSAIDs are contraindicated or should be used with caution in patients at risk for postsurgical bleeding and in those with aspirin-induced asthma, renal insufficiency, preexisting ulcer disease, and CHF.[18]

It is unfortunate that some surgeons withhold perioperative administration of NSAIDs because of animal studies that detected an increase in wound-site bleeding and impaired bone remodeling. It should be mentioned that those investigations used relatively high doses of NSAIDs for prolonged treatment periods. In clinical settings, patient safety may be maintained by limiting dose size and dose duration (24 to 36 hours). In addition, emerging local-acting, injectable NSAIDs, such as DepoNSAID, may provide local activity while even further minimizing concerns regarding systemic toxicity.

Coxibs have also been advocated for multimodal analgesia. In a large randomized trial, Sinatra and coworkers[19] reported that cotreatment with rofecoxib for 5 days following abdominal surgery not only reduced pain intensity scores and opioid consumption

TABLE 5.3 — Multimodal Analgesics Advocated for Acute Pain Management

Agent	Mode of Action	Dose	Efficacy	Safety
NSAIDs	COX-2 inhibition	IV: ketorolac 15-30 mg q6h IV: ibuprofen 800 mg q6h	30% reduction in pain intensity and opioid dose	Wound site and GI bleeding,[a] renal toxicity
Acetaminophen	GABA inhibition, serotonergic interaction	PO: 650 mg q6h IV: 1000 mg q6h	20% to 30% reduction in pain intensity and opioid dose, IV >PO	Hepatotoxicity
α-Agonists	Enhanced monoamine-mediated analgesia	Patch (clonidine): 0.1 mg/24h Epidural (Duraclon): 20-30 mcg/h Dexmedetomidine: 0.1 mcg/h	Opioid-sparing reduction in pain intensity; epidural >patch	Hypotension[b], bradycardia
Ketamine	Nonselective NMDA antagonism	1 mg/kg/h infusion	≥30% reduction in pain and opioid dose	Hallucinations, confusion[c]
Gabapentinoids	α2δ ion channel blockade	Gabapentin 600 mg tid Pregabalin 100 mg bid	Opioid-sparing, reduced hyperalgesia and neuropathic symptoms	Sedation[d]

Local anesthetics	Nerve-conduction blockade, infiltration	Ropivacaine 0.2% infiltration Bupivacaine 0.1% to 0.25% infiltration EXPAREL (bupivacaine liposome injectable suspension)1.3% infiltration[f]	Opioid-sparing, significant decrease in pain intensity	Neurotoxicity, cardiotoxicity
Tricyclic anti-depressants	Norepinephrine reuptake inhibitor	Imipramine 25 mg every day	Reduction in neuropathic pain	Sedation[e], dry mouth
Dual-acting analgesics	μ-opioid agonist and norepinephrine reuptake inhibition	Tapentadol 50-100 mg q6h	Equipotent to oxycodone 10 mg with less GI adverse events	Sedation

[a] Ketorolac should not be administered preoperatively.
[b] Epidural clonidine may precipitate acute hypotension in elderly patients and those with ongoing surgical bleeding.
[c] Analgesia and CNS effects are dose dependent; use the lowest dose possible.
[d] Adjust dose carefully in renal failure patients
[e] Best if administered in the evening.
[f] EXPAREL (bupivacaine liposomal injectable suspension); typical infiltration dose is 8 to 20 cc of 1.3%.

FIGURE 5.1 — Targets for Multimodal Analgesics

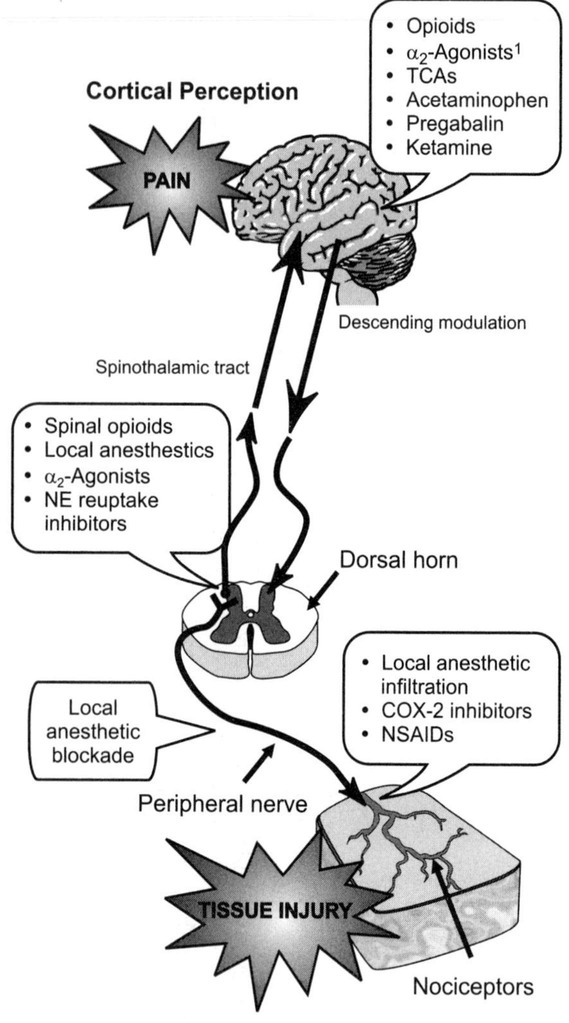

Key: NE, norepinephrine; NSAID, nonsteroidal anti-inflammatory drug; TCA, tricyclic antidepressant.

[1] Gottschalk A, Smith DS. *Am Fam Physician*. 2001;63(10):1979-1984.

but also resulted in significantly less sedation and more rapid return of bowel function. Although rofecoxib has since been withdrawn from the market, similar benefits may be anticipated following coadministration of celecoxib (Celebrex). Celecoxib is only available as an oral tablet (200 mg). It can be given 2 to 3 hours prior to induction of anesthesia and will provide 12 hours of anti-inflammatory and noxious suppression with minimal effects on platelet function. Its disadvantage is that it cannot be used in patients who have not been advanced to an oral liquid diet.

A second, very important method of suppressing transduction and initial noxious transmission is infiltration of local anesthetic into the site of injury.[20] Intermediate duration of action solutions of 0.25% to 0.5% bupivacaine (Marcaine) or 0.5% ropivacaine (Naropin) injected SC and into fascia can block noxious signaling and pain intensity for 8 to 12 hours. Unfortunately, with these shorter-acting agents, pain returns as the block wanes, and patients must be reminded to take other pain relievers as soon as they notice slight increases in levels of discomfort. Until recently, one of the biggest disadvantages of available agents is their relatively short duration of action. Newer agents, such as EXPAREL (bupivacaine liposome injectable suspension), have been shown to be safe and effective in reducing pain with an attendant reduction in opioid use, in both soft tissue and boney surgeries, up to 72 hours after local administration. Pressure-powered "pain buster" pumps may be employed to continuously infuse dilute solutions of bupivacaine into the wound site and can provide more prolonged and effective pain relief as well. These pumps are expensive, and catheters used for infusion into the wound may become dislodged and ineffective. Single-dose infiltration of EXPAREL (bupivacaine liposome injectable suspension) has been demonstrated to provide up to 72 hours of pain relief in several surgical models.[21] This preparation is expected to play a major role in surgeon-managed multimodal analgesia and benefit fast-track opioid-reduction treatment plans.

■ Conduction

Pain signals from peripheral nociceptors travel primarily along small, myelinated A and unmyelinated C fibers, which synapse in the spinal cord. Local anesthetic infiltration and neural blockade may be used to effectively block noxious signaling in peripheral nerves and to reduce pain intensity and overall analgesic requirements. Anesthesiologists employ ultrasound or nerve stimulation techniques either to more efficiently and reliably administer single boluses of local anesthetic or to guide catheter placement for continuous infusions.

Single-bolus perineural injections of ropivacaine 0.5% or bupivacaine 0.5% may provide ≥8 to 16 hours of effective analgesia. Continuous infusions of either bupivacaine or ropivacaine offer more prolonged relief but require placement of a perineural catheter. Once the catheter is placed, infusions can be maintained for up to 96 hours during the inpatient recovery period. Catheters may be placed into nerve sheaths or nerve plexi to control severe pain associated with hand, arm, shoulder, knee, and ankle procedures. In some institutions, selected patients may be discharged with catheters in place and infusions maintained with pressure-powered pumps. Infusate solutions of bupivacaine and ropivacaine may be diluted as low as 0.2% to 0.25% to selectively block small pain fibers while sparing the larger sensory and motor fibers. Infusions are delivered at rates between 8 and 14 mL/hour, depending upon patient habitus and pain complaint. Continuous infusions of bupivacaine 0.25% into the femoral nerve sheath provide pain relief that is superior to IV-PCA with fewer AEs and facilitate return of function (greater knee flexion) in patients recovering from total knee replacement surgery.[22,23] Catheters may also be placed in the paravertebral space for relief of thoracic and abdominal postsurgical pain. Transabdominal aponeurosis blocks may be provided for pain relief following cesarean section, hysterectomy, and prostatectomy.

■ Spinal Transmission

An ideal target for multimodal suppression of noxious signaling is the synapse between the primary nociceptive fiber and the second-order transmission cell in the spinal cord. Analgesics administered via spinal and epidural needles or catheters, as well as parenteral and oral routes, can bind to endogenous receptors and enhance local and descending inhibitory mechanisms.

Local Mechanisms

Local mechanisms include inhibitory interneurons that release enkephalins and activate pre- and postsynaptic opioid receptors. Spinal administration of morphine, fentanyl, or hydromorphone allows a relatively large number of molecules to bind these receptors, resulting in powerful and prolonged analgesia. Continuous epidural infusions of fentanyl or hydromorphone can be maintained for up to 96 hours.[24,25] The addition of ultradilute concentrations of bupivacaine (0.02%) or ropivacaine (0.1%) to the infusion provides spinal neural blockade and additional analgesic benefits. While catheter placement is invasive, epidural infusions of an opioid plus a local anesthetic provide the most efficient and effective form of pain control for thoracic and abdominal surgeries, including colectomy, as well as for orthopedic total knee replacement.

A prolonged-duration epidural morphine preparation (DepoDur) that incorporates liposomal technology, similar to EXPAREL (bupivacaine liposome injectable suspension) is available for severe abdominal and lower extremity surgical pain. DepoDur offers the advantages of:

- Single-dose administration
- Does not require catheter placement or infusion pumps
- Can provide up to 48 hours of pain relief.

Its major drawbacks are annoying dose-related nausea, vomiting, and pruritus, which can be minimized by reducing the recommended 10-mg to 15-mg dose to

7.5 mg or less and supplementing with NSAIDs, acetaminophen, and other multimodal analgesics.

Unfortunately, many patients who could benefit from epidural analgesia are denied this option due to changes in surgical preference for anticoagulation. Catheters cannot be placed in patients treated with low molecular weight heparinoids or warfarin (Coumadin).[26]

Ketamine is a nonselective NMDA receptor antagonist that can suppress the sensitization of second order spinal neurons. Once activated by noxious transmitters, the NMDA receptor is responsible for continuous cell firing ("wind-up"), the development of secondary sensitization and changes in neural connections that may lead to persistent pain.[27,28] Low-dose IV ketamine infusions (0.1 mg/kg/hr) antagonize NMDA-induced changes and provide effective augmentation of analgesia.[27] Such therapy is generally well tolerated and is not associated with the hallucinations and dysphoria seen with high-dose administration of ketamine. Ketamine infusions are particularly useful in patients who are intolerant to opioids and in others who have significant degrees of opioid tolerance or hyperalgesia.[27,28]

Descending Inhibition

Descending inhibition is mediated by enkephalinergic and noradrenergic neurons in the brainstem that send descending axons to the spinal cord that normally inhibit pain transmission. IV and oral opioids, as well as α-adrenergic blockers such as clonidine and dexmedetomidine, bind to endogenous opioid or α-adrenergic receptors and enhance endogenous analgesia.[29,30] Clonidine (Catapres) transdermal patch offers a noninvasive convenient way to administer the drug at a rate of 0.2 mg/24 hours. Its analgesic benefits are useful in patients intolerant of opioids and are best appreciated when the patch is applied prior to surgery. Epidural solutions of clonidine (Duraclon) offer greater potency and are as effective as opioids in suppressing spinal pain transmission.[31] One advantage of epidural clonidine is that, when compared with opioids, it is less likely to cause nausea and vomiting. For this reason, it is widely used for pediatric pain management. Epidural clonidine should only be prescribed for healthy adults as it is associated with hypotension, particularly in debilitated and hypovolemic patients.[31]

Nucynta (Tapentadol) is a central-acting analgesic that has dual actions in the spinal cord and other areas of the brain. It provides multimodal analgesia by activating spinal opioid receptors and also by enhancing α-adrenergic–mediated analgesia. Tapentadol blocks the norepinephrine reuptake protein on terminal endings of descending axons, thereby increasing concentrations of norepinephrine and enhancing α-adrenergic–mediated pain suppression. Clinical studies indicate that tapentadol provides efficacy that is comparable to that of oxycodone with significantly less nausea vomiting, constipation, and pruritus.[32]

Other drugs that can be used to enhance spinal and supraspinal α-adrenergic analgesia include TCAs and serotonin-norepinephrine reuptake inhibitors (SNRIs).[33,34] These agents provide antineuropathic effects and are useful in patients with a nerve injury component (eg, thoracotomy, mastectomy, amputation) to their postsurgical pain.[33] They also provide antidepressant benefits for patients unable to cope with severe pain or those with poor outcomes following onocologic surgery. In contrast to the delayed onset of antidepressant activity, the onset of TCA-based analgesia is fairly rapid (24 hours). Since TCAs can be sedating, they are best administered prior to sleep.

■ Spinal Reflexes

Hyperalgesic spinal motor responses to peripheral injury increase skeletal muscle tone in dermatomes at and adjacent to the site of trauma. Increasing muscle spasm and accumulation of lactic acid result in increased sensitization and pain.[35] Opioids have minimal effect on hyperalgesic muscular spasm but can diminish associated pain. Administration of skeletal muscle relaxants, including judicious doses of diazepam and lorazepam, can inhibit muscle spindle activity and reduce pathologic spasm. By breaking the cycle of pain causing muscle spasm and increasing spasm causing increasing pain, patients benefit from greater comfort and reduced opioid dose. It should be remembered that coadministration of benzodiazepines and other muscle relaxants will increase central sedation; therefore doses of other central-acting agents, particularly opioids, should be reduced.[36]

■ Cortical Perception

Pain is perceived in the sensory motor and limbic cortex. A number of central-acting analgesics can be administered to blunt pain perception, including opioids, gabapentinoids, acetaminophen, certain NSAIDs, TCAs, and SNRIs. Opioids, including morphine, hydromorphone, oxycodone, and fentanyl, suppress pain intensity and suffering but have less effect on pain localization. In multimodal regimens, opioid dosing is restricted and employed primarily for breakthrough pain.[37]

Acetaminophen (*N*-acetyl-para-aminophenol, APAP) provides a central analgesic effect that is mediated through activation of descending serotonergic pathways, although the precise mechanism by which this occurs remains unclear.[38] Oral and rectal forms of acetaminophen are erratically absorbed in postsurgical settings yet provide measurable analgesic effects and should be used in patients tolerating oral diets.[38] IV acetaminophen (Ofirmev), which was FDA approved for use in the United States in 2010, and provides improved pain relief and opioid-sparing comparable to ketorolac.[39] When used as directed, the safety profile of IV acetaminophen relative to opioids and NSAIDs suggests that it may be better suited for general and orthopedic surgical patients. It has no effect on respiratory drive, mental status, gastric mucosa, renal function, or rates of bleeding.

Anticonvulsant analgesics, including gabapentin (Neurontin) and pregabalin (Lyrica), were initially developed to control chronic neuropathic pain.

However, several studies have shown this class of medications can also suppress aspects of acute surgical pain.[40,41] Although their exact mechanism of action remains unknown, gabapentinoids are believed to bind and modulate $\alpha_2\delta$ voltage-dependent calcium channels and thereby stabilize sensitized neuronal membranes. Gabapentin blocks the sensitization phase of nociception and reduces opioid dose requirements in patients with neuropathic and osteogenic postsurgical pain. Doses of 600 mg gabapentin or 100 mg pregabalin may be administered 2 hours preoperatively and continued as needed in patients tolerating oral diets.[41] Gabapentinoids should be considered for use in patients undergoing surgery in which peripheral nerves are transected and in all postsurgical patients complaining of neuropathic pain.

Differences between opioid monotherapeutic approaches to pain management and multimodal analgesia are presented in **Figure 5.2**.

Preemptive Analgesia

A second pain-management strategy that has gained renewed attention is preemptive analgesia. It was first employed in the early nineteenth century by the American surgeon GW Crile who, prior to incision, applied Novocaine to the surgical site in patients anesthetized with ether. In the late 1980s, Wall and later Kehlet, a general surgeon, proposed the concept of "preemptive preoperative analgesia," suggesting that analgesic intervention is most effective when made in advance of the pain stimulus rather than in reaction to it.[42,43] Preoperative administration of NSAIDs, local anesthetic infiltration, and local anesthetic neural blockade–produced analgesic effects that long outlasted the pharmacologic duration of the agents/techniques employed. One of the first clinical trials designed to detect benefits of pre- vs postsurgical neural blockade was performed by Ringrose and Cross in 1984.[44] They noted that patients treated with femoral

FIGURE 5.2 — Opioid Monotherapy vs Multimodal Analgesia

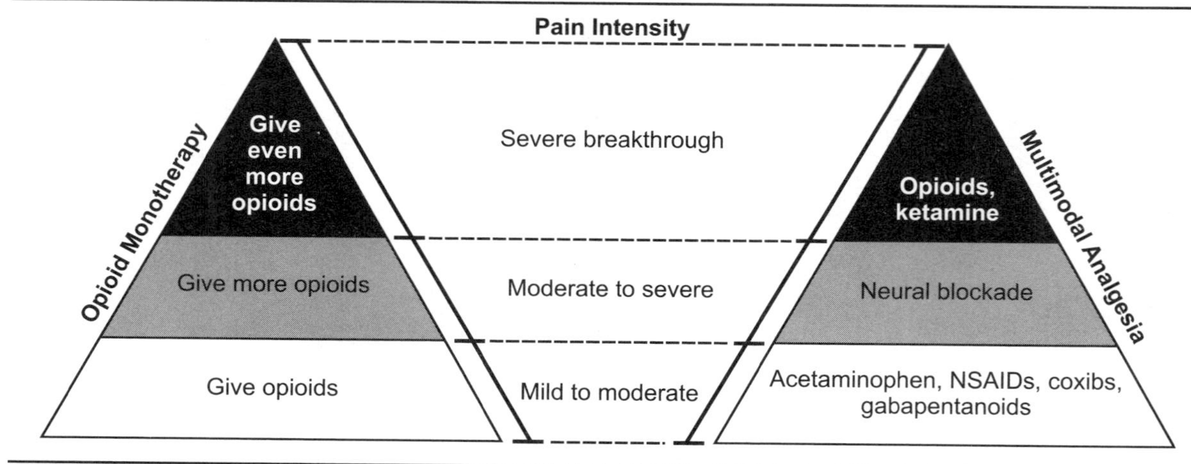

nerve block prior to arthroscopic knee surgery required 50% less opioid analgesic during the first 24 hours of recovery than individuals receiving a similar block at completion of the procedure. One drawback to providing local anesthetic prior to the surgical procedure is their relatively short duration of action. With the recent availability of local anesthetic formulations that can last for days, this drawback may be eliminated.

Based on these observations, other investigators have studied and reported good efficacy for preemptive administration of analgesics to block transmission of noxious stimuli and thereby preclude the cascade of events that leads to peripheral and central sensitization.[45-47] In contrast to other analgesics, preemptive administration of IV or oral opioids is not associated with improved postsurgical analgesia and is not recommended.[48] Several studies have demonstrated that preoperative opioid loading is associated with acute tolerance development and may also precipitate opioid-induced hyperalgesia (OIH). Both conditions lead to increased opioid dose requirements. OIH is also associated with paradoxic increases in the intensity of postsurgical pain.

It is now recognized that benefits associated with preemptive analgesia are gained only when preincisional therapy is seamlessly maintained well into the postsurgical period.[45,47] Perioperative analgesia is ideally maintained for 24 to 48 hours for outpatient surgery and 96 hours or longer for more invasive inpatient procedures. It includes:

- Preoperative dosing prior to surgical incision
- Continued dosing during anesthesia
- Postsurgical maintenance of therapy
- Adequate analgesic prescription following hospital discharge (**Figure 5.3**).

While the majority of clinical studies have concentrated on improving postsurgical pain and acute disability, preemptive analgesia may also provide longer-term convalescent-rehabilitative benefits and

FIGURE 5.3 — Perioperative Analgesia

Recognition that surgical pain results from:
- Trauma during surgical dissection
- Postoperative inflammation and aggravation of tissue injury during movement

Multimodal analgesics should be given continuously throughout the perioperative operative period

- Preoperatively
- Intraoperatively
- Postoperatively
- Postdischarge

either prevent or minimize the severity of persistent pain syndromes.[48-50] Patients recovering from back-fusion surgery, in which donor bone is taken from the iliac crest, may develop chronic periosteal pain that persists for months to years after the operation. Infusion of bupivacaine via an iliac crest catheter attenuates the intensity of acute postsurgical pain and appears to minimize development of chronic sensitivity.[48]

Neuralgias, phantom limb pain, and deafferentation syndromes are common after amputation. Preemptive analgesia provided by perioperative epidural conduction blockade can prevent the development of chronic stump and phantom limb pain in patients recovering from below the knee amputation.[51]

Conclusion

The use of opioid monotherapy as a method to achieve better pain control is precluded by dose-limiting side effects.[4] In contrast, multimodal anesthesia provides a rational stepwise approach to improved analgesic efficacy while minimizing the side effects associated with any one class of drug. The increased availability of injectable nonopioid analgesics and improvements in regional analgesia have dramatically increased interest and application of multimodal analgesia.

A number of new nonopioid analgesics and analgesic adjuncts are in development and will further compliment perioperative multimodal analgesia and reduce the need for opioids. Although a significant body of positive evidence has been published, large-scale and longer-term studies are required to determine if multimodal analgesia is cost-effective and whether it results in improvements in objective outcomes above and beyond reductions in opioid use.

REFERENCES

1. Practice guidelines for acute pain management in the perioperative setting. A report by the American Society of Anesthesiologists Task Force on Pain Management, Acute Pain Section. *Anesthesiology*. 1995;82(4):1071-1081.
2. Peters CL, Shirley B, Erickson J. The effect of a new multimodal perioperative anesthetic regimen on postoperative pain, side effects, rehabilitation, and length of hospital stay after total joint arthroplasty. *J Arthroplasty*. 2006;21(6 suppl 2):132-138.
3. Franklin PD, Karbassi JA, Li W, Yang W, Ayers DC. Reduction in narcotic use after primary total knee arthroplasty and association with patient pain relief and satisfaction. *J Arthroplasty*. 2010;25(6 suppl):12-16.
4. Oderda GM, Said Q, Evans RS, et al. Opioid-related adverse drug events in surgical hospitalizations: impact on costs and length of stay. *Ann Pharmacother*. 2007;41(3):400-406.
5. Wheeler M, Oderda GM, Ashburn MA, Lipman AG. Adverse events associated with postoperative opioid analgesia: a systematic review. *J Pain*. 2002;3(3):159-180.
6. Schug SA, Zech D, Grond S. Adverse effects of systemic opioid analgesics. *Drug Saf*. 1992;7(3):200-213.
7. Gan TJ, Lubarsky DA, Flood EM, et al. Patient preferences for acute pain treatment. *Br J Anaesth*. 2004;92(5):681-688.
8. Kehlet H, Dahl JB. The value of "multimodal" or "balanced analgesia" in postoperative pain treatment. *Anesth Analg*. 1993;77(5):1048-1056.
9. Kehlet H, Wilmore DW. Multimodal strategies to improve surgical outcome. *Am J Surg*. 2002;183(6):630-641.
10. Joshi GP. Multimodal analgesia techniques and postoperative rehabilitation. *Anesthesiol Clin North America*. 2005;23(1): 185-202.
11. White PF. Multimodal analgesia: its role in preventing postoperative pain. *Curr Opin Investig Drugs*. 2008;9(1):76-82.
12. Elia N, Lysakowski C, Tramèr MR. Does multimodal analgesia with acetaminophen, nonsteroidal antiinflammatory drugs, or selective cyclooxygenase-2 inhibitors and patient-controlled analgesia morphine offer advantages over morphine alone? Meta-analyses of randomized trials. *Anesthesiology*. 2005;103(6):1296-1304.
13. Vane JR, Botting RM. Mechanism of action of nonsteroidal anti-inflammatory drugs. *Am J Med*. 1998;104(3A):2S-8S.

14. Cashman JN. The mechanisms of action of NSAIDs in analgesia. *Drugs*. 1996;52(suppl 5):13-23.

15. Seybold VS, Jia YP, Abrahams LG. Cyclo-oxygenase-2 contributes to central sensitization in rats with peripheral inflammation. *Pain*. 2003;105(1-2):47-55.

16. Toradol prescribing information. http://www.drugs.com/pro/ketorolac-tromethamine.html. Accessed December 1, 2011.

17. Caldolor (intravenous ibuprofen) [package insert] http://www.caldolor.com/pdfs/Caldolor_Full_Prescribing_Information.pdf. Accessed December 1, 2011.

18. Pham K, Hirschberg R. Global safety of coxibs and NSAIDs. *Curr Top Med Chem*. 2005;5(5):465-473.

19. Sinatra RS, Boice JA, Loeys TL, et al. Evaluation of the effect of perioperative rofecoxib treatment on pain control and clinical outcomes in patient recovering from gynecologic abdominal surgery: a randomized, double-blind, placebo-controlled clinical study. *Reg Anesth Pain Med*. 2006;31(2):134-142.

20. Ritchey RM. Optimizing postoperative pain management. *Cleve Clin J Med*. 2006;73(suppl 1):S72-S76.

21. Pacira Pharmacueticals. Exparel. Data on file. 2011.

22. Capdevila X, Barthelet Y, Biboulet P, Ryckwaert Y, Rubenovitch J, d'Athis F. Effects of perioperative analgesic technique on the surgical outcome and duration of rehabilitation after major knee surgery. *Anesthesiology*. 1999;91(1):8-15.

23. Hebl JR, Dilger JA, Byer DE, et al. A pre-emptive multimodal pathway featuring peripheral nerve block improves perioperative outcomes after major orthopedic surgery. *Reg Anesth Pain Med*. 2008;33(6):510-517.

24. Grass JA. Fentanyl: clinical use as postoperative analgesic–epidural/intrathecal route. *J Pain Symptom Manage*. 1992;7(7):419-430.

25. Dabu-Bondoc S, Franco S, Sinatra R. Neuraxial analgesia with hydromorphone, morphine, and fentanyl: dosing and safety guidelines. In: Sinatra R, de-Leon-Casasola O, Ginsberg B, Viscusi E, eds. *Acute Pain Management*. New York, NY: Cambridge University Press; 2009:230-244.

26. Horlocker TT, Wedel DJ, Rowlingson JC, et al. Regional anesthesia in the patient receiving antithrombotic or thrombolytic therapy: American Society of Regional Anesthesia and Pain Medicine Evidence-Based Guidelines (Third Edition). *Reg Anesth Pain Med*. 2010;35(1):64-101.

27. De Kock M, Lavand'homme P, Waterloos H. 'Balanced analgesia' in the perioperative period: is there a place for ketamine? *Pain*. 2001;92(3):373-380.

28. Elia N, Tramèr MR. Ketamine and postoperative pain–a quantitative systematic review of randomised trials. *Pain*. 2005;113 (1-2):61-70.

29. Segal IS, Jarvis DJ, Duncan SR, White PF, Maze M. Clinical efficacy of oral-transdermal clonidine combinations during the perioperative period. *Anesthesiology*. 1991;74(2):220-225.

30. Jeffs SA, Hall JE, Morris S. Comparison of morphine alone with morphine plus clonidine for postoperative patient-controlled analgesia. *Br J Anaesth*. 2002;89(3):424-427.

31. Milligan KR, Convery PN, Weir P, Quinn P, Connolly D. The efficacy and safety of epidural infusions of levobupivacaine with and without clonidine for postoperative pain relief in patients undergoing total hip replacement. *Anesth Analg*. 2000; 91(2):393-397.

32. Guay DR. Drug treatment of paraphilic and nonparaphilic sexual disorders. *Clin Ther*. 2009;31(1):1-31.

33. Brander VA, Stulberg SD, Adams AD, et al. Predicting total knee replacement pain: a prospective, observational study. *Clin Orthop Relat Res*. 2003;(416):27-36.

34. O'Connor AB, Noyes K, Holloway RG. A cost-effectiveness comparison of desipramine, gabapentin, and pregabalin for treating postherpetic neuralgia. *J Am Geriatr Soc*. 2007;55(8): 1176-1184.

35. Chou R, Peterson K, Helfand M. Comparative efficacy and safety of skeletal muscle relaxants for spasticity and musculoskeletal conditions: a systematic review. *J Pain Symptom Manage*. 2004;28(2):140-175.

36. Valium [package insert]. Ontario: Hoffmann-LaRoche Limited; 1998.

37. White PF. The changing role of non-opioid analgesic techniques in the management of postoperative pain. *Anesth Analg*. 2005;101(5 suppl):S5-S22.

38. Toms L, McQuay HJ, Derry S, Moore RA. Single dose oral paracetamol (acetaminophen) for postoperative pain in adults. *Cochrane Database Syst Rev*. 2008;(4):CD004602.

39. Sinatra RS, Jahr JS, Reynolds LW, Viscusi ER, Groudine SB, Payen-Champenois C. Efficacy and safety of single and repeated administration of 1 gram intravenous acetaminophen injection (paracetamol) for pain management after major orthopedic surgery. *Anesthesiology*. 2005;102(4):822-831.

40. Tiippana EM, Hamunen K, Kontinen VK, Kalso E. Do surgical patients benefit from perioperative gabapentin/pregabalin? A systematic review of efficacy and safety. *Anesth Analg*. 2007;104(6):1545-1556.

41. Ho KY, Gan TJ, Habib AS. Gabapentin and postoperative pain–a systematic review of randomized controlled trials. *Pain*. 2006;126(1-3):91-101.

42. Wall PD. The prevention of postoperative pain. *Pain*. 1988;33 (3):289-290.

43. Dahl JB, Kehlet H. The value of pre-emptive analgesia in the treatment of postoperative pain. *Br J Anaesth*. 1993;70(4):434-439.

44. Ringrose NH, Cross MJ. Femoral nerve block in knee joint surgery. *Am J Sports Med*. 1984;12(5):398-402.

45. Woolf CJ, Chong MS. Preemptive analgesia–treating postoperative pain by preventing the establishment of central sensitization. *Anesth Analg*. 1993;77(2):362-379.

46. Bromley L, Richmond C, Brandner B, Woolf C. Pre-emptive analgesia. *Anaesthesia*. 1995;50(2):176-177.

47. Gottschalk A, Smith DS. New concepts in acute pain therapy: preemptive analgesia. *Am Fam Physician*. 2001;63(10):1979-1984.

48. Angst MS, Clark JD. Opioid-induced hyperalgesia: a qualitative systematic review. *Anesthesiology*. 2006;104(3):570-587.

49. Visser E. Chronic post-surgical pain: epidemiology and clinical implications for acute pain management. *Acute Pain*. 2006;8:73-81.

50. Perkins FM, Kehlet H. Chronic pain as an outcome of surgery. A review of predictive factors. *Anesthesiology*. 2000;93(4): 1123-1133.

51. Bach S, Noreng MF, Tjéllden NU. Phantom limb pain in amputees during the first 12 months following limb amputation, after preoperative lumbar epidural blockade. *Pain*. 1988;33(3):297-301.

6

Opioid-Mediated Analgesia

by Raymond S. Sinatra, MD, PhD

Introduction

Opioids are a class of central-acting analgesics that provide powerful dose-dependent pain relief. They have and still remain the therapeutic foundation for the management of moderate to severe postsurgical pain.[1-3] Opioids include compounds:

- With variable pharmacokinetics
- With no cardiac or hepatorenal toxic effects
- With no ceiling effect for achievable pain relief
- That are available for oral, parenteral, and neuraxial administration.

Opioid Pharmacology

Opioids interact with specific transmembrane G protein–coupled binding sites termed opioid receptors. These receptors are located primarily in spinal dorsal horn, central gray matter, limbic cortex, and other regions of the CNS that process the suffering and emotional aspects of pain perception.[1-3] Naturally occurring opiates (eg, morphine) and synthetic opioids (eg, oxycodone, hydrocodone) have structural or chemical characteristics that permit binding and activation of opioid receptors, resulting in powerful analgesia (**Figure 6.1**). Four opioid receptor subtypes, designated as μ, κ, δ, and σ have been characterized.[1-4]

μ Receptors mediate supraspinal analgesia and euphoria, as well as respiratory depression, nausea and vomiting, bowel hypomotility, and physical and psychological dependence.[1,2] κ Receptors are responsible for spinal analgesia, visceral analgesia, and sedation,

FIGURE 6.1 — Classification of Naturally Occurring, Semisynthetic, and True Synthetic Opioid Families

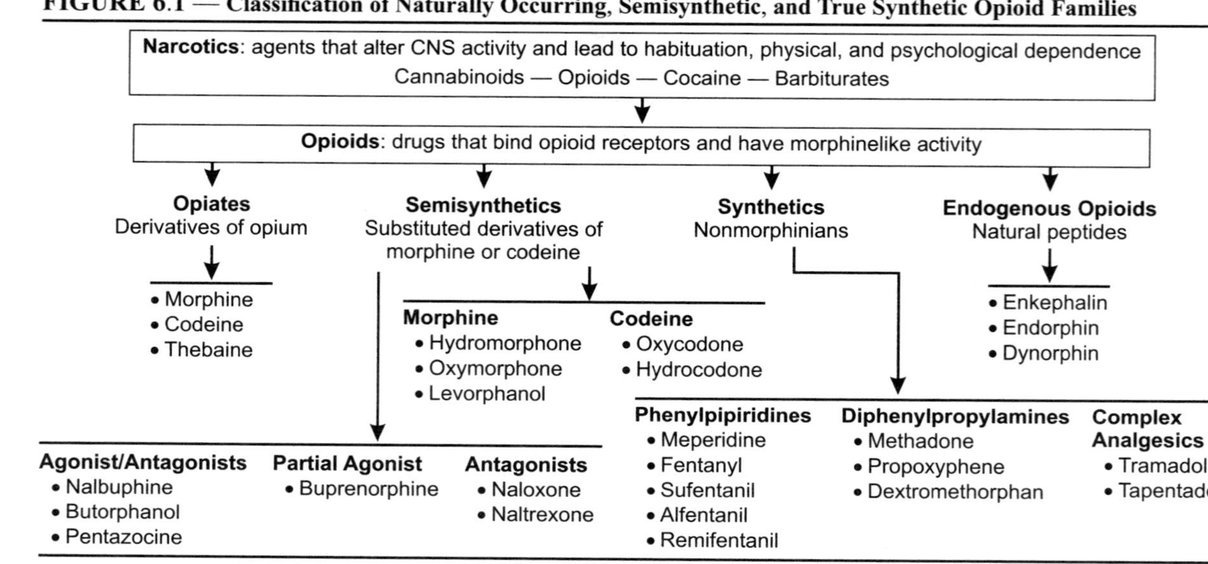

but have minimal effect on respiration.[1-3] σ Receptors are believed to be responsible for opioid-related dysphoria, hallucinations, and confusion.

Based on binding specificity, opioids are classified as either[1-4]:

- Agonists
- Partial agonists
- Mixed agonist-antagonists
- Complete antagonists.

Opioid agonists include compounds such as morphine, hydromorphone, or fentanyl that bind receptors with moderate-to-high affinity and are capable of producing a maximal analgesic response. Partial agonists, such as buprenorphine, have high affinity at μ receptors but activate them incompletely. The analgesic efficacy curve of partial agonists is bell shaped, such that low doses provide increasing levels of analgesia to a point after which additional doses either do not increase pain relief or slightly diminish it.[1-3] This "analgesic ceiling effect" restricts their use to patients with mild-to-moderate pain (**Figure 6.2**). Antagonists such as naloxone and naltrexone bind to all receptor subtypes with high affinity but do not activate the receptor. Antagonists competitively block the activity of agonists by preventing or displacing their binding to the receptor.

Opioid analgesic onset is determined by the ability of an agonist to enter the CNS and distribute into gray matter where receptors are primarily localized.[1-3,5] Opioid potency, or the amount of drug required to achieve an analgesic effect, is closely related to the lipophilicity and intrinsic efficacy of the agonist. As a rule, highly lipophilic opioids, such as fentanyl, have significantly greater potency than hydrophilic agents such as morphine.[1,3,5,6] Analgesic duration is related to several factors, including receptor dissociation kinetics, and both plasma and CSF elimination kinetics. Pharmacologic correlates of opioid effects are presented in **Table 6.1**.

FIGURE 6.2 — Opioid Dose-Response Curves

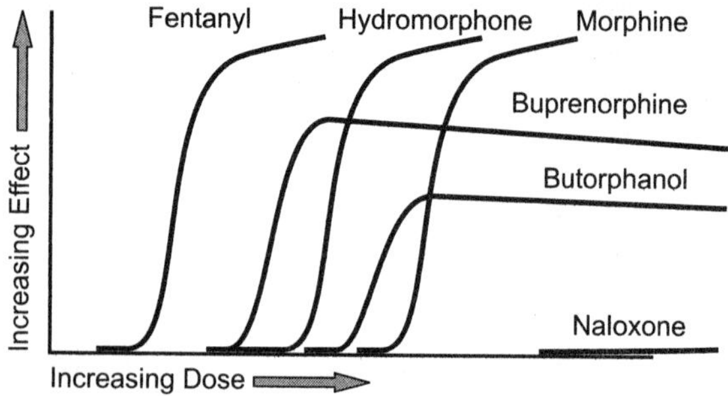

These curves illustrate the potency and efficacy of various opioid analgesics. Potent agonists, such as fentanyl, require the lowest dose to achieve the maximal analgesic effect. Morphine achieves the maximal effect but requires a considerably greater number of molecules to be administered. Mixed agonist-antagonists and partial agonists such as buprenorphine are either more or less potent than morphine; however, they cannot achieve the maximal effect despite increases in dose. This ceiling effect in analgesic efficacy limits their ability to control moderate-to-severe pain. The antagonist naloxone has no analgesic efficacy.

Tolerance and Hyperalgesia

Continued patient exposure to opioid analgesics leads to tolerance development and clinical manifestations, such as physical dependence. Tolerance is defined as the progressive increases in dose required to maintain a desired pharmacologic effect and is characterized by a shift to the right in the classic dose-response curve.[1-3,7,8] This physiologic adaptation is observed in patients prescribed opioids for pain relief, as well as in those abusing this class of drug. Physical dependence is a normal and commonly observed phenomenon in opioid-tolerant patients. Upon abrupt discontinuation of opioids, parasympathetic tone is markedly increased,[1,2,7,8] and patients experience unpleasant withdrawal symptoms including sweating, shaking, cramping, and diarrhea.

TABLE 6.1 — Pharmacologic Correlates of Opioid Activity

Potency
• High lipid solubility
Onset
• Low degree of ionization
• High CNS penetration
• High receptor affinity
Duration
• High water solubility (CSF trapping)
• High receptor binding kinetics
• Low hepatic/renal clearancc
• Active metabolites
• Large volume of distribution
Safety
• μ Receptor specificity
• Lack of active or toxic metabolites
Efficacy
• Multiple receptor specificity
• High receptor affinity
• High intrinsic efficacy

Psychological dependence includes drug-seeking behavior and use for purposes other than pain control. Addiction is a term describing an extreme form of psychological dependence where patients demonstrate craving, compulsive drug seeking, and continued use despite harm. Surgeons and their patients should recognize that unlike physical dependence, opioid addiction is rarely observed in patients suffering moderate-to-severe postsurgical pain.[9]

A second clinical alteration observed in patients treated with opioids is termed "opioid-induced hyperalgesia" (OIH).[10] This phenomenon is characterized by paradoxic increases in pain intensity and the development of new pain complaints in response to increasing administration of opioid analgesics. OIH is most often observed in tolerant patients but has also been observed in naïve individuals. Excitatory effects of opioid metabolites (eg, morphine-3-glucoronide, hydromorphone-3-glucoronide) may also play a role in the development and progression of OIH. Treatment of OIH includes discontinuation or dose reduction of the offending opioid, switching to a different agonist (opioid rotation) such as methadone, and use of adjuvants such as ketamine.[10]

Parenteral Opioid Therapy

Since oral analgesics are poorly tolerated during the immediate postsurgical period, parenteral (IV, IM, and SC) opioids are commonly prescribed for surgical pain management. There are several situations in which parenteral opioids may be employed:

- IV-PCA
- Nurse-administered IV bolus
- IV/IM opioids administered by the clock or PRN.

■ Administration Using IV-PCA

IV-PCA allows patients to titrate opioids in amounts necessary to reduce pain intensity to a tolerable level.[11] Opioids commonly employed for IV-PCA include morphine and hydromorphone, with fentanyl reserved for highly tolerant or allergic patients. A loading dose of opioid is usually administered for immediate pain control prior to initiation of patient-initiated bolus doses. Bolus doses generally range from 1 mg to 1.5 mg for morphine or 0.2 mg to 0.3 mg for hydromorphone. A bolus lockout interval or minimum delay between doses is usually 6 to 8 minutes. A basal infusion equivalent to 1 bolus dose administered over a 1-hour interval may be provided to opioid-tolerant patients and others with very severe pain. Patients prefer PCA to parenteral analgesic techniques as it offers greater control for their pain management and that they do not have to worry about receiving too much or too little drug.[12]

PCA systems work under a number of assumptions, the first being that opioid side effects occur at higher CNS concentrations than those needed to produce analgesia.[11] While extremely high opioid doses could theoretically eliminate all pain (but with unacceptable levels of respiratory depression), an adequate level of analgesia usually represents a compromise between tolerable pain and troublesome side effects. A second assumption is that pain intensity is rarely constant. Postsurgical pain is intensified by movement and physical therapy, and seems to have a circadian rhythm, with increasing pain at night.[11,12] Nighttime pain is especially problematic since that is when adequate staffing may be limited and physicians are least available.

6

Two common reasons why patients become dissatisfied and fail with PCA include:

- Inadequate analgesia
- Excessive nausea/vomiting.

Patients must be trained to treat pain before the stimulus becomes overwhelming. For example, incremental boluses should be administered prior to physical therapy or any form of movement that might increase discomfort. They must also understand that PCA may never completely eliminate their pain, and that if side effects are experienced, they should ask for medication or call the nurse or pain service to reduce their dose. They should not stop using the PCA device and suffer in silence. Finally, concerned relatives or visitors should never push the PCA button for the patient![13,14]

The safety and efficacy of IV-PCA requires motivated, alert, and well-informed patients, trained clinical and pharmacy staff, and specific order sets. Problems associated with IV-PCA include patient overuse of drug, and the fact that the infusion pump, IV lines, and power cables often interfere with patient mobility.[11] To reduce these potential drawbacks, IV-PCA is generally reserved for patients who are on NPO orders and it should be restricted to the first 24 to 36 hours following surgery. Reduced-dose IV-PCA morphine (0.5 mg bolus dose) or hydromorphone (0.1 mg bolus dose) may be effective when employed with multimodal analgesic adjuvants or as a supplement for continuous regional nerve block or longer-acting local anesthetic infiltration techniques.

■ Nurse-Administered IV Bolus

Nurse-administered IV bolus doses per patient request (PRN) are useful for individuals advancing from IV-PCA or epidural opioid-based analgesia who have moderate-to-severe discomfort but have yet to tolerate oral diets. Parenteral dosing is of particular importance in patients who are nauseated or vomiting, who might not absorb oral agents.

■ IV/IM Opioids Administered by the Clock or PRN

Several subsets of patients, including the elderly, the cognitively impaired, and overly dependent individuals, are poor candidates for IV-PCA and may achieve better pain control with IV/IM opioids administered by the clock or PRN.[11,15] These patients might also benefit from nonopioid adjuvants. In these individuals, PRN requests and total parenteral dose administered during early postsurgical intervals may be used to calculate follow-up oral analgesic dosing. Opioid-dependent patients with significant tolerance development may require both baseline chronic opioid therapy (eg, methadone, controlled-release oxycodone), as well as IV-PCA or parenteral opioid infusions for acute surgical pain.[8]

Oral Analgesic Dosing

Oral administration offers a convenient, noninvasive, and cost-effective method of controlling acute pain that should always be considered in patients who continue to experience moderate-to-severe discomfort. Oral opioids, including morphine, hydrocodone, and oxycodone, and compounded preparations containing acetaminophen, aspirin, and ibuprofen can provide effective relief, depending upon pain intensity levels and drug tolerability. Orally administered morphine and meperidine are poorly absorbed and undergo significant enterohepatic metabolism.[1,2] When compared with parenteral dosing, onset is delayed, duration is less predictable and dose requirements are increased.

Short-acting oral opioids agents, such as morphine immediate release (IR), hydrocodone IR, hydromorphone IR, oxycodone IR, and oxymorphone IR, may be favored initially because they are better tolerated and easier to titrate.[2,15,16] Oxycodone and hydrocodone are more reliably absorbed than morphine.[15] These agents are best employed in opioid-naïve patients recovering from uncomplicated procedures that require relatively limited durations of treatment.

6

Short-acting opioids are characterized by a rapid rise and fall in serum opioid levels, whereas serum levels of sustained-release opioids increase slowly to therapeutic levels, remain there for an extended period, then decline slowly.[17] Opioid toxicity and adverse events are most likely to occur at these peak serum levels. Sustained-release opioid preparations, including morphine (MS Contin), oxycodone (Oxycontin), and oxymorphone (Opana ER), while not primarily indicated for surgical pain management, offer several advantages, including less frequent administration intervals, avoidance of peak-and-trough plasma levels and greater analgesic uniformity.[17,18] These preparations provide 8 to 12 hours of pain relief and are best suited for patients suffering chronic pain or prolonged postsurgical pain.

An additional opioid preparation that may be considered for patients who cannot tolerate oral analgesics but continue to experience brief episodes of severe pain is the fentanyl oralet (Actiq and other generic equivalents). Fentanyl oralet releases between 100 mcg and 400 mcg of fentanyl within 15 minutes, with high bioavailability.[19]

Less-potent opioid analgesics, such as tramadol and codeine, may be prescribed to patients recovering from procedures associated with mild to moderate pain. A compounded form of tramadol (Ultracet) provides greater effectiveness than tramadol alone. Ultracet is an oral multimodal analgesic containing tramadol plus acetaminophen, approved for the short-term management of acute pain.[20] A newer and more powerful "dual-acting" analgesic, tapentadol (Nucynta), activates μ-opioid receptors and also inhibits norepinephrine reuptake. Although its analgesic efficacy is equivalent to that of oxycodone, it has a better tolerability profile, causing less nausea, vomiting, constipation, and puritus.[21,22] Oral and parenteral opioids employed for postsurgical pain management are detailed in *Chapter 7*.

Neuraxial Opioids

Neuraxial administration of opioid analgesics into the spinal (intrathecal) or epidural space can provide powerful pain control in patients recovering from a variety of surgical procedures. Following spinal or epidural administration, opioid molecules traverse the CSF and bind to receptors in the dorsal horn, effectively blocking pain transmission at the first synapse in the CNS. Epidural and spinally administered opioids provide greater analgesic potency than similar doses administered parenterally.[23,24] Morphine (Astamorph, Duramorph) was first to receive Food and Drug Administration (FDA) approval for spinal use and remains the most widely used opioid for spinal analgesia.[23] A single spinal dose (0.2 mg to 0.75 mg) is commonly utilized for control of pain following thoracic, abdominal, pelvic, and lower extremity surgery.[23] In general, analgesic onset is appreciated after 30 to 60 minutes, peak effect at 90 to 120 minutes, and duration of effect is prolonged, ranging from 12 to 24 hours. Surgeons should understand that spinal morphine doses are only 1/10 to 1/20th of the 24-hour parenteral morphine dose while providing superior pain relief. In addition, spinal morphine is basically a single-dose technique and cannot match the duration and analgesic uniformity of continuous epidural opioid infusions.

Continuous epidural infusions and patient-controlled epidural analgesia (PCEA) offer high analgesic efficacy and patient satisfaction, with lower dose requirements than IV-PCA or IV boluses of parenteral opioids. Analgesic effects can be maintained for a prolonged period of time (24 to 96 hours), depending upon the site and invasiveness of the surgical procedure. Epidural doses of morphine are associated with a high incidence of pruritus and delayed-onset respiratory depression.[23] Hydromorphone and fentanyl have become the epidural opioids of choice as they:

- Have rapid onset
- Can easily be titrated to analgesic effect
- Have greater tolerability and safety.[24-28]

6

Epidural solutions of hydromorphone (10-20 mcg/mL) and fentanyl (5 mcg/mL) are generally infused at 6 to 16 mL/hour, depending upon the location of the epidural catheter and the number of dermatomes involved in the surgery.[24-27] Infusions via thoracic epidural catheters are recommended for chest and upper abdominal procedures, while lumbar catheters may be used for pelvic and lower extremity surgeries. Patient-controlled bolus doses of 2 to 4 mL every 6 to 10 minutes may be added to continuous epidural infusions to better control pain with procedures and movement. Finally, the effectiveness of epidural opioids may be further improved by the addition of dilute solutions of bupivacaine or ropivacaine.[27,28] It should be recognized that the addition of local anesthetics often results in sensory/motor and sympathetic blockade and hypotension in volume-depleted patients. Agents and doses recommended for continuous epidural infusions and epidural PCA are outlined in **Table 6.2**.

Epidural- and spinal-administered opioids are associated with a number of annoying and occasionally serious adverse effects, including pruritus, nausea, urinary retention, somnolence, and respiratory depres-

TABLE 6.2 — Dosing Guidelines for Epidural Opioid Infusions and PCA[a,b]

Opioid	Site of Administration	Continuous Infusion Technique	PCA Technique	Adjunctive Therapy
Morphine	Lumbar catheters: incisions below T8 Thoracic catheters: upper abdominal and thoracic surgery	2-4 mg bolus followed by infusion (40 mcg/mL); Lumbar catheters: 6-12 mL/h Thoracic catheters: 4-8 mL/h	2-4 mg bolus followed by infusion (40 mcg/mL); Lumbar catheters: 6-8 mL/h Thoracic catheters: 2-6 mL/h PCEA bolus dose 1-2 mL q15min	IV ketorolac or ibuprofen, oral celecoxib, IV-acetaminophen; add epidural bupivacaine (0.05%-0.1%)
Hydromorphone	Lumbar catheters: incisions below T10 Thoracic catheters: upper abdominal and thoracic surgery	0.5-1.5 mg bolus followed by infusion (10-20 mcg/mL); Lumbar catheters: 8-14 mL/h Thoracic catheters: 4-8 mL/h	0.5-1.5 mg bolus followed by infusion (10-20 mcg/mL); Lumbar catheters: 6-10 mL/h Thoracic catheters: 4-6 mL/h PCEA bolus dose 1-3 mL q6-8min	IV ketorolac or ibuprofen, oral celecoxib, IV-acetaminophen; add epidural bupivacaine (0.05%-0.1%)

Fentanyl	Lumbar catheters: incisions below T12 Thoracic catheters: almost everything else	50-100 mcg bolus followed by infusion (4 mcg/mL); Lumbar catheters: 8-14 mL/h Thoracic catheters: 4-8 mL/h	50-100 mcg bolus followed by infusion (4-5 mcg/mL); Lumbar catheters: 6-10 mL/h Thoracic catheters: 4-6 mL/h PCEA bolus dose 1-3 mL q6min	IV ketorolac or ibuprofen, oral celecoxib, IV-acetaminophen; add epidural bupivacaine (0.05%-0.1%)

[a] Dependent on age, physical status, height, extent of surgical dissection, degree of opioid tolerance, etc.
[b] Unless contraindicated.

6

sion.[24,28] Pruritus and nausea are the most common side effects associated with epidural or spinal opioids; however, respiratory depression is the most feared complication.[24,28] Mild elevations in $PaCO_2$ are commonly observed with effective epidural analgesia. The incidence of clinically significant respiratory depression or arrest ranges between 0.1% and 0.4%.[24] Morbidly obese patients and those with obstructive sleep apnea and chronic obstructive pulmonary disease are at highest risk for severe respiratory compromise.[24,28] In addition to pulse oximetry, vigilant nursing observation and documentation of inadequate respiratory effort, slow respiratory rate, or unusual somnolence represent the best form of monitoring.[24,28] Prophylactic naloxone infusions (400 mcg/L) at 100-125 mL/hour have been advocated to reduce the risk of opioid-induced respiratory depression in elderly or debilitated patients while maintaining effective analgesia.[24,28] Naloxone infusions effectively reduce the incidence and severity of other adverse effects, including pruritus, nausea, and urinary retention.

Contraindications to spinal opioid analgesia include spinal fracture, infection at the insertion site, septicemia, coagulopathy, and treatment with low-molecular weight heparinoids. Concern has been raised about the safety of using anticoagulant-based prophylaxis of deep venous thrombosis (DVT) with regional anesthesia in patients undergoing surgery.[29] In December 1997, the FDA issued an advisory letter about the potential risk of epidural hematoma in patients receiving regional (spinal or epidural) anesthesia and low molecular weight heparin (LMWH). The American Society of Regional Anesthesia (ASRA) issued guidelines with respect to the safe use of anticoagulants in patients to be treated with neuraxial analgesia.[30] The use of LMWH with spinal and epidural analgesia is safe as long as published guidelines and recommendations from experienced clinical authorities are observed.

Opioid-Related Adverse Events

In settings of acute pain, most opioid-related AEs are transient and tend to resolve with ongoing treatment.[1-3] Common AEs associated with parenteral and orally administered opioids and their active metabolites include nausea, vomiting, sedation, pruritus, and constipation.[31] In sensitive individuals, the incidence and severity of these AEs may be so annoying and distressing that patients self-limit or discontinue opioid dosing and suffer poor pain control.[31,32] Patients recovering from colorectal and gynecologic surgery are generally at risk for opioid-induced bowel dysfunction and ileus, mandating that such therapy be supplemented with stool softeners, bulk laxatives, and occasional enemas.

Most opioid-related AEs are dose dependent, which is why it is important to initiate therapy with the lowest effective dose and to utilize a multimodal analgesic approach. Some opioid-related AEs are often treated symptomatically, eg, by prescribing an antiemetic for nausea or laxatives and/or a peripheral μ antagonist for constipation.[1,3,32] Other side effects, such as sedation and pruritus, are typically addressed by decreasing the opioid dose rather than by treating the symptom. In addition to dose reductions, other strategies that can be employed to minimize opioid-related AEs include changing the route of administration, switching to a different opioid, or providing adjuvant analgesic therapy.[32]

Variability in Opioid Response

Opioids tend to have a highly variable response in individual patients. A therapeutic failure with one opioid agonist does not necessarily mean that the patient will fail to respond to others. Pharmacokinetic and pharmacodynamic variables and other interindividual genetic variations can result in clinically measurable differences in analgesic efficacy and adverse effect profile between opioid agonists[33,34] (**Table 6.3**). The concept of incomplete cross tolerance describes the unexpectedly improved effectiveness or tolerability of a newly prescribed agonist when compared with equivalent doses of others that the patient has found unacceptable. In recent years, over 20 polymorphisms of the μ-opioid receptor gene (OPRM1) have been identified.[35] In a clinical trial that evaluated patients with opioid receptor polymorphisms of gene 118, those homozygous for allele GG self-administered significantly more morphine and incurred more AEs during the first 48 hours following knee surgery than those homozygous for the AA allele (homozygous AA 25 mg, heterozygous AG 26 mg, homozygous GG 40 mg).[36]

TABLE 6.3 — Patient Variability in Opioid Response

- μ-Opioid receptor polymorphisms
- Opioid tolerance
- Genetic alterations in opioid metabolism (CYP-450)
- Incomplete cross-tolerance
- Extremes in patient age
- Exposure to drugs that compete for metabolic enzymes
- Exposure to drugs that increase CNS depression
- Patient comorbidity (hepatic failure, CNS lesions, renal failure)

Conclusion

Opioids will continue to play a major role in post-surgical pain management for the considerable future. Existing parenteral and oral analgesics offer effective pain relief, although no agonist can provide the optimal combination of high efficacy and low side effect profile for all patients. For the near term, novel delivery systems for existing opioids and the ongoing development of dual-acting compounds will provide new tools to help facilitate surgeon- and anesthesiologist-based pain management. Increasing knowledge regarding opioid receptor polymorphisms may permit patients to be screened and treatment plans developed preoperatively, thereby ensuring that the optimal agonist can be administered perioperatively.

REFERENCES

1. Reisine T, Pasternak G. Opioid analgesics and antagonists. In: Goodman LS, Gilman A, eds. *The Pharmacologic Basis of Therapeutics.* 9th ed. New York, NY: Macmillan;1997.
2. Gutstein HB, Akil H. Opioid analgesics. In: Hardman JG, Limbird LE, Gilman AG, eds. *Goodman & Gilman's The Pharmacological Basis of Therapeutics.* 10th ed. New York, NY: McGraw-Hill; 2002:569-619.
3. Pasero C, Portenoy RK, McCaffery M. Opioid analgesics. In: McCaffery M, Pasero C. *Pain Clinical Manual.* St. Louis, MO: Mosby Inc; 1999:161-299.
4. Sinatra R. Opioid analgesics in primary care: challenges and new advances in the management of noncancer pain. *J Am Board Fam Med.* 2006;19:165-177.
5. Beecher HK. Pain in men wounded in battle. *Ann Surg.* 1946; 123(1):96-105.
6. Way WL, Fields HL, Schumaker MA. Opioid analgesics. In: Katsung BG, ed. *Basic and Clinical Pharmacology.* 9th ed. New York, NY: Lange Medical Books/McGraw-Hill; 2004.
7. Nestler EJ, Aghajanian GK. Molecular and cellular basis of addiction. *Science.* 1997;278(5335):58-63.
8. Mitra S, Sinatra RS. Perioperative management of acute pain in the opioid-dependent patient. *Anesthesiology.* 2004;101(1):212-227.
9. Portenoy RK, Farrar JT, Backonja MM, et al. Long-term use of controlled-release oxycodone for noncancer pain: results of a 3-year registry study. *Clin J Pain.* 2007:23(4):287-299.
10. Angst MS, Clark JD. Opioid-induced hyperalgesia: a qualitative systematic review. *Anesthesiology.* 2006;104(3):570-587.
11. Etches RC. Patient-controlled analgesia. *Surg Clin North Am.* 1999;79(2):297-312.
12. Chumbley GM, Hall GM, Salmon P. Why do patients feel positive about patient-controlled analgesia? *Anaesthesia.* 1999;54(4):386-389.

13. Eade DM. Patient-controlled analgesia–eliminating errors. *Nurs Manage*. 1997;28(6):38-40.

14. Herrick IA, Ganapathy S, Komar W, et al. Postoperative cognitive impairment in the elderly. Choice of patient-controlled analgesia opioid. *Anaesthesia*. 1996;51(4):356-360.

15. Marco CA, Plewa MC, Buderer N, Black C, Roberts A. Comparison of oxycodone and hydrocodone for the treatment of acute pain associated with fractures: a double-blind, randomized, controlled trial. *Acad Emerg Med*. 2005;12(4):282-288.

16. Ross FB, Smith MT. The intrinsic antinociceptive effects of oxycodone appear to be kappa-opioid receptor mediated. *Pain*. 1997;73(2):151-157.

17. Stambaugh JE, Reder RF, Stambaugh MD, Stambaugh H, Davis M. Double-blind, randomized comparison of the analgesic and pharmacokinetic profiles of controlled- and immediate-release oral oxycodone in cancer pain patients. *J Clin Pharmacol*. 2001;41(5):500-506.

18. Opana ER (oxymorphone hydrochloride) extended release tablets [package insert]. Chadds Ford, PA: Endo Pharmaceuticals Inc; September 2010.

19. Actiq (fentanyl citrate) oral transmucosal lozenge [package insert]. Frazer, PA: Cephalon, Inc; July 2011.

20. Simpson DM, Messina J, Xie F, Hale M. Fentanyl buccal tablet for the relief of breakthrough pain in opioid-tolerant adult patients with chronic neuropathic pain: a multicenter, randomized, double-blind, placebo-controlled study. *Clin Ther*. 2007;29(4):588-601.

21. Sinatra RS, Sramcik J. Tramadol: its use in pain management. *Anesthesiol Clin North America*. 1998;2:53-69.

22. Daniels S, Casson E, Stegmann JU, et al. A randomized, double-blind, placebo-controlled phase 3 study of the relative efficacy and tolerability of tapentadol IR and oxycodone IR for acute pain. *Curr Med Res Opin*. 2009;25(6):1551-1561.

23. Hartrick C, Van Hove I, Stegmann JU, Oh C, Upmalis D. Efficacy and tolerability of tapentadol immediate release and oxycodone HCl immediate release in patients awaiting primary joint replacement surgery for end-stage joint disease: a 10-day, phase III, randomized, double-blind, active- and placebo-controlled study. *Clin Ther*. 2009;31(2):260-271.

24. Wong C. *Spinal and Epidural Anesthesia*. New York, NY: McGraw-Hill; 2006:75-110.

25. Ginosar Y, Riley ET, Angst MS. The site of action of epidural fentanyl in humans: the difference between infusion and bolus administration. *Anesth Analg*. 2003;97(5):1428-1438.

26. Curatolo M, Petersen-Felix S, Scaramozzino P, Zbinden AM. Epidural fentanyl, adrenaline and clonidine as adjuvants to local anaesthetics for surgical analgesia: meta-analyses of analgesia and side-effects. *Acta Anaesthesiol Scand*. 1998;42(8): 910-920.

27. Grass JA. Fentanyl: clinical use as postoperative analgesic–epidural/intrathecal route. *J Pain Symptom Manage*. 1992;7(7): 419-430.

28. Dabu-Bondoc S, Franco S, Sinatra R. Neuraxial analgesia with hydromorphone, morphine, and fentanyl: dosing and safety guidelines. In: Sinatra RS, de-Leon-Casasola OA, Ginsberg B, Viscusi ER, eds. *Acute Pain Management*. New York, NY: Cambridge University Press; 2009:230-244.

29. Tam NL, Pac-Soo C, Pretorius PM. Epidural haematoma after a combined spinal-epidural anaesthetic in a patient treated with clopidogrel and dalteparin. *Br J Anaesth*. 2006;96(2):262-265.

30. Horlocker TT, Wedel DJ, Rowlingson JC, et al. Regional anesthesia in the patient receiving antithrombotic or thrombolytic therapy: American Society of Regional Anesthesia and Pain Medicine Evidence-Based Guidelines (Third Edition). *Reg Anesth Pain Med*. 2010;35(1):64-101.

31. Wheeler M, Oderda GM, Ashburn MA, Lipman AG. Adverse events associated with postoperative opioid analgesia: a systematic review. *J Pain*. 2002;3(3):159-180.

32. Sinatra RS, Torres J, Bustos AM. Pain management after major orthopaedic surgery: current strategies and new concepts. *J Am Acad Orthop Surg*. 2002;10(2):117-129.

33. Galer BS, Coyle N, Pasternak GW, Portenoy RK. Individual variability in the response to different opioids: report of five cases. *Pain*. 1992;49(1):87-91.

34. Mogil JS. The genetic mediation of individual differences in sensitivity to pain and its inhibition. *Proc Natl Acad Sci U S A*. 1999 ;96(14):7744-7751.

35. Uhl GR, Sora I, Wang Z. The mu opiate receptor as a candidate gene for pain: polymorphisms, variations in expression, nociception, and opiate responses. *Proc Natl Acad Sci U S A*. 1999;96(14):7752-7755.

36. Chou WY, Yang LC, Lu HF, et al. Association of mu-opioid receptor gene polymorphism (A118G) with variations in morphine consumption for analgesia after total knee arthroplasty. *Acta Anaesthesiol Scand*. 2006;50(7):787-792.

7 Oral and Parenteral Opioids for Postsurgical Pain Management

by Raymond S. Sinatra, MD, PhD

Introduction

Opioid analgesics are advocated and widely prescribed for the management of moderate-to-severe postsurgical pain.[1-4] In recent years, opioids have been increasingly advocated as analgesics for breakthrough pain in patients treated with regional anesthesia and multimodal analgesia rather than administered around the clock as primary monotherapy.[1] In the immediate postsurgical period, patients are usually treated with PCA or caregiver-administered parenteral opioids, titrated to the intensity of the pain complaint. As soon as patients are able to tolerate a liquid diet, they should be advanced to orally administered opioids, which can be continued during the convalescent and rehabilitative periods following surgery.[1,3,4] Morphine and oxycodone are primarily used in inpatient settings; hydromorphone, hydrocodone, and most recently tapentadol, offer therapeutic alternatives for patients experiencing inadequate pain control or intolerable adverse effects.[1-4]

The advantages and disadvantages of parenteral and oral opioids are presented in **Table 7.1**.

Parenteral Opioids

■ Morphine

Parenterally administered morphine remains the standard of care for control of acute pain following surgical and traumatic injuries.[2-5] Ten mg to 15 mg of parenteral morphine, in divided doses, is generally

TABLE 7.1 — Oral and Intravenous Opioid Analgesics

Benefits

- Rapid onset of analgesia for moderate, severe, and very severe pain
- Highly effective analgesia (no analgesic dose ceiling)
- Selective analgesia:
  - Reductions in pain suffering
  - Minimal effects on pain localization
- No effects on key organs:
  - Cardiac
  - Renal
  - Hepatic
  - Hemostatic safety
- Multiple agents and routes of administration are available
- Relatively inexpensive (morphine, oxycodone)

Drawbacks

- Annoying side effects:
  - Nausea
  - Pruritus
  - Sedation
  - Constipation
- Clinically significant effects:
  - Ileus
  - Bowel obstruction
  - Severe vomiting
  - Confusion
  - Dysphoria
- Life-threatening effects:
  - Airway obstruction
  - Respiratory depression
  - Respiratory arrest
- Social effects:
  - Dose escalation
  - Physical dependence
  - Diversion and abuse
  - Addiction
- May be expensive (sustained-release opioids, oral buccal preparations)

recommended as a starting dose for moderate-to-severe surgical pain in patients weighing >50 kg.[1-3] Onset of analgesia with IV morphine is noted within 5 to 15 minutes, while duration ranges from 2 to 4 hours, depending upon dose administered.[3,5] Small doses of IV morphine (2 mg to 3 mg every 1 to 2 hours) may be administered for breakthrough pain in patients treated with continuous regional blockade.[1] Parenteral boluses of morphine may also be administered to patients who were initially treated with IV-PCA morphine or epidural analgesia, yet remain NPO.

Morphine is associated with clinically significant dose-dependent adverse effects.[2-6] These include annoying side effects such as nausea, vomiting, and pruritus, and serious, occasionally life-threatening side effects such as excessive sedation and respiratory depression. Oral and IV doses of morphine release histamine, which may precipitate hypotension and bronchospasm.[2-4,6] Morphine also increases smooth muscle tone and may induce or exacerbate biliary, tubular, and ureteral colic. Like other opioid agonists, morphine's effect on respiratory drive will increase $PaCO_2$ and may raise intracranial pressure.[2-4] Morphine's principal metabolite (morphine-6-glucoronide) has significant potency and is primarily excreted in the urine.[7] For this reason, it should not be administered to patients with acute renal failure.[2,3]

■ Hydromorphone (Dilaudid)

Parenteral doses of hydromorphone provide rapid and powerful control of postsurgical pain.[3,5,6,8] Following slow IV administration, analgesia is noted in 2 to 5 minutes, peak effect in 10 to 15 minutes, and duration ranges from 2 to 3 hours.[2,4,6,8,9] Hydromorphone is less hydrophilic than morphine, and its ability to penetrate the blood-brain barrier (BBB) is greater. It is approximately five times as potent as morphine and offers greater efficacy for patients with very severe pain. Hydromorphone also provides a good replacement for patients allergic or intolerant to morphine. Inpatients treated 24 to 72 hours with IV-PCA hydromorphone, who remain NPO or are just tolerating oral diet, may be transitioned to IV bolus doses (1 mg to 2 mg) of hydromorphone every 3 hours. The high concentration of hydromorphone solutions (2 to 4 mg/mL) also allow it to be administered SC with minimal patient discomfort.

Except for a ketone substitution, hydromorphone's chemical structure and molecular weight are similar to those of morphine.[2,3] Hydromorphone has a side effect profile similar to that of other opioids, including dose-dependent nausea, sedation, and respiratory depression. It appears to have a lower incidence of pruritus and excessive sedation than morphine.[3,4]

Hydromorphone is primarily metabolized by hepatic glucuronidation.[2,8,9] Drug accumulation and exaggerated effects can be expected in settings of hepatic and renal failure. Its principal metabolite (hydromorphone-6-glucoronide) is inactive. For this reason, hydromorphone may be cautiously administered to patients with renal failure.[10]

■ Oxymorphone (Opana IV)

Oxymorphone is a highly potent opioid analgesic that has been available for >40 years.[11] It is approved for surgical pain management and is currently available in a 1-mg vial. Oxymorphone has approximately ten times greater potency than morphine. Its onset to peak effect is more rapid than that of morphine and its overall analgesic efficacy is superior.[12,13] Analgesic onset is noted within 5 minutes and the duration of effect can last 3 to 4 hours.[13,14] IV oxymorphone should be reserved for patients experiencing very severe pain in the PACU and surgical care units. Rather than spending considerable time titrating doses of morphine, 1 mg to 2 mg of IV oxymorphone can rapidly establish an effective level of analgesia for patients recovering from painful procedures and others with a high-grade opioid tolerance.[15]

Meperidine (Demerol)

IV and IM doses of meperidine were often prescribed for surgical pain management. Over the last 10 years, such therapy has fallen from favor because of potential neurologic adverse events. Meperidine's renally cleared metabolite (normeperidine) accumulates in patients with diminished kidney function and can provoke tremors, myoclonus, and seizures.[2,3,15]

Meperidine has a parenteral potency that is one tenth that of morphine, with a duration of effect that is only two thirds as long. Doses of 100 mg to 120 mg may be required every 2 hours if given IV and every 3 hours if administered IM.[2,3,15] Meperidine was initially developed as an anticholinergic, has smooth muscle relaxant effects, and is effective in controlling visceral cramping and colicky pain. Doses ranging from 75 mg to 100 mg may be administered to patients recovering from laproscopic cholecystectomy, ovarian and tubular procedures, and bladder surgery.[15] In some patients, low doses of meperidine (50 mg to 100 mg) are more effective than morphine in controlling visceral discomfort associated with acute pancreatitis and cholelithiasis.[3,15]

Methadone (Dolophine)

Parenteral doses of methadone may be considered for patients with opioid tolerance and others suffering severe acute pain that is poorly responsive to morphine and hydromorphone. In acute pain settings, methadone doses of 0.25 to 0.3 mg/kg employed as monotherapy provide effective analgesia for up to 12 hours. Patients generally require little to no supplementation with IV-PCA opioids.[16-18] Following lower abdominal surgery, patients treated with parenteral methadone 20 mg intraoperatively followed by PRN doses in PACU reported less pain and need for supplemental opioids than others treated with equivalent doses of morphine.[17] In a very large (3954) inpatient series, methadone was effective for patients suffering prolonged and very painful surgical- and medical-related acute pain.[19]

Methadone may also be employed as an adjuvant or as primary therapy. Adjuvant doses of ≤0.1 mg/kg every 12 hours provides useful augmentation of the analgesic effects provided by a primary opioid such as hydromorphone or oxycodone.[20] Methadone is also advocated for patients suffering nerve injuries and neuropathic pain, as well as individuals who are highly opioid dependent or opioid hyperalgesic.[20,21]

Methadone is associated with opioid-related side effects, including sedation, confusion, nausea, and vomiting, but unlike morphine and meperidine, it does not release histamine. Methadone blocks potassium channels expressed in myocardial cells. Therapeutic plasma levels are associated with prolongation of the QT interval and may initiate or exacerbate torsades de pointes and reentry arrhythmias.[3,4,22] A screening EKG may be necessary to evaluate the QT interval when methadone doses exceed 60 mg/day.[22]

■ Fentanyl (Sublimaze)

Fentanyl is employed in hypotensive patients or those with well-documented allergies to naturally occurring or semisynthetic opioids.[2-4,23] Fentanyl is associated with minimal effects on cardiac output or blood pressure. Because of its hemodynamic stability, it is safer than morphine for use in patients with clinically significant cardiac and cerebral disease.[2,3,23]

Doses of 50 mcg to 200 mcg are commonly administered to patients recovering from ambulatory surgery and provide rapid pain relief. Similar doses offer useful analgesia for patients requiring closed reductions and dressing changes.[3,23]

IV infusions of fentanyl (0.5 to 5 mcg/kg/hour) may be used for sedation and pain control in ventilated or hemodynamically unstable patients. Infusion rates may be increased or diminished in response to inadequate pain control or to minimize adverse events. In addition, bolus doses of fentanyl (25 mcg to 50 mcg) or hydromorphone (0.5 mg to 1 mg) may be administered for breakthrough pain.[23]

■ DepoDur (EREM)

A single-dose, extended-release epidural morphine (EREM) drug called DepoDur may be a step toward a longer-acting morphine analogue. DepoDur has been found to have a duration of action up to 48 hours with long-lasting analgesia in the absence of large systemic concentrations of opioids, as well as better patient activity levels. Several studies have shown that EREM produces long-term pain relief.[24] Epidural anesthesia has been used for colorectal resections, showing beneficial outcomes for both laparoscopic and open techniques.[25]

Side effects of EREM can be treated with opioid antagonists. The elderly are particularly sensitive to the effects of EREM and require close perioperative monitoring. It was shown that the elderly treated with 15 mg of EREM had equivalent fentanyl usage as younger patients treated with 20 mg of EREM.[24]

Oral Opioids

■ Morphine

Oral morphine remains the world standard for surgical pain management. Clinically, it has high analgesic potency, a slow onset-to-peak effect, and an intermediate duration of activity.[1,2,4] Morphine's delayed onset of analgesia has been related to the fact that it has difficulty penetrating the BBB.[2,3,26] Morphine is poorly absorbed from the GI tract and doses are generally three times higher than that required parenterally.[26,27]

Typical doses for postsurgical pain management are 20 mg to 40 mg every 4 to 6 hours. Morphine elixir may be better tolerated than oral tablets in patients who have just been advanced to oral diet.[5,6,26]

■ Oxycodone (Roxicodone, Oxycontin)

Oxycodone is a semisynthetic μ- and κ-receptor agonist that is commonly prescribed in the United States for postsurgical pain.[3,5,26,28,29] Oxycodone has high oral bioavailability because of rapid GI absorption and limited enterohepatic metabolism. In clinical practice, oxycodone does not release significant amounts of histamine and is associated with less sedation than equivalent doses of morphine.[2,3] Oxycodone, like codeine and hydrocodone, is primarily metabolized through microsomal CYP3A4 and/or CYP2D6 pathways.[2-4] Coadministration of medications that interact with these pathways may affect the plasma levels of oxycodone, resulting in reduced analgesia or adverse events. Up to 12% of oral oxycodone is demethylated and converted to oxymorphone, a highly potent opioid agonist.[2,28,29]

Oxycodone is a versatile analgesic available as either an oral tablet, elixir (OxyIR), or compounded with acetaminophen. Typical doses for surgical pain management are 5 mg to 15 mg every 4 to 6 hours. Compounds containing oxycodone provide greater analgesic effects than oxycodone alone and include those containing acetaminophen (Percocet, Lortab) or ibuprofen (Combunox).[30,31] Controlled-release (CR) oxycodone preparations (eg, Oxycontin) are available and offer prolonged (12 hours) and uniform analgesia, avoiding troughs of effect observed with IR oxycodone. When converting surgical patients from IV-PCA morphine to controlled-release oxycodone, calculate the prior 24-hour dose of morphine, then multiply by 1.5. One half of that amount is then given twice daily, with additional IR oxycodone 5 mg provided if requested (**Table 7.2**).[32]

■ Hydrocodone-Acetaminophen Compound (Vicodin, Lortab)

Hydrocodone is a μ-selective opioid agonist that is commonly prescribed for inpatient and outpatient surgical pain management. This semisynthetic derivative of codeine provides greater potency and analgesic efficacy, as well as improved tolerability, than the parent compound.[2,26,28,32] Although the oral analgesic potency of hydrocodone is equivalent to that of oxycodone, many clinicians in the United States consider it to be a weaker drug with lower abuse potential.

TABLE 7.2 — Conversion Factors for Estimating the Initial Daily Dose of Oral Oxycodone CR in the Postsurgical Setting[a]

Prior IV Opioid	Conversion Factor
Morphine	1.5
Meperidine	0.2
Hydromorphone	10
Fentanyl	200-300

[a] The initial oxycodone CR dose was calculated according to the formulas:

Prior IV opioid (mg/day) × conversion factor = oral oxycodone CR dose (mg/day)

Oral oxycodone CR dose (mg/day)/2= initial oral oxycodone CR dose (mg q12h)

7

Compounded hydrocodone plus acetaminophen tablets, up to 15 mg and total 300 mg hydrocodone per day, are less controlled (schedule III) than other semisynthetic opioids and generally do not require triplicate prescriptions. This lower level of regulation, together with hydrocodone's reliability in relieving moderate-to-severe pain, explains why it is so widely prescribed by surgical caregivers.[26,28,32] Hydrocodone undergoes hepatic O-demethylation by CYP2D6 into the more potent opioid hydromorphone, which is eventually glucoronidated and excreted in urine.[2,3] Patients who are extensive CYP2D6-hydrocodone metabolizers report greater analgesic benefits than poor metabolizers.[2]

■ Hydromorphone (Dilaudid)

Hydromorphone (Dilaudid) is a semisynthetic, μ-selective opioid agonist developed >80 years ago and used for treatment of moderate to severe pain. It has an oral analgesic potency five to six times greater than morphine, and its onset of effect is more rapid.[2,3,33,34]

Oral doses of hydromorphone are associated with less histamine release than morphine and are less likely to precipitate hypotension and bronchoconstriction.[2,3] In the United States, hydromorphone is often substituted for morphine in postsurgical settings. It is particularly useful in patients with severe pain unresponsive to morphine, and in those who have had safe and effective pain control with IV-PCA or IV bolus doses of hydromorphone. It is also employed in individuals with high-grade opioid tolerance and patients suffering adverse events with oral hydrocodone or oxycodone.[3,26] Hydromorphone is available as oral tablets and as an oral elixir.

■ Oxymorphone (Opana IR, Opana ER)

Oxymorphone is a semisynthetic μ-selective opioid agonist.[2,11] Oxymorphone has poor GI absorption and high enterohepatic metabolism. For this reason, its oral potency is only one tenth that of IV oxymorphone, and three times that of oral morphine.[2,35] Oxymorphone is primarily metabolized by hepatic glucoronidation and not by CYP-450 enzymes.[2,35] It neither inhibits nor induces CYP-450 pathways. These properties may offer clinical advantages over oxycodone and codeine for patients coadministered other medications metabolized by this pathway.[2,11,35]

Oxymorphone IR (Opana IR) is available as an oral tablet for moderate-to-severe acute pain.[35] The analgesic effectiveness, safety, and tolerability of this preparation have been demonstrated in several postsurgical pain trials.[35,36] Oxymorphone is also available as a sustained-release analgesic that provides a reliable 12-hour duration of effect (Opana ER).[35] Sustained-release oxymorphone is not indicated for surgical pain unless it is expected to be very severe and of prolonged duration.[35]

■ Tapentadol (Nucynta)

Tapentadol was FDA approved in 2009 and is the first new oral analgesic for moderate to severe acute pain in >25 years. Tapentadol is a potent, dual-acting analgesic that combines central μ-opioid receptor agonism with monoamine reuptake inhibition to suppress pain transmission. Tapentadol offers analgesic efficacy comparable to classic opioids but with unexpectedly improved GI tolerability.[37] The efficacy and safety of tapentadol IR compared with 10 mg to 15 mg oxycodone IR have been evaluated in several placebo-controlled postsurgical pain trials.[37,38] These trials demonstrated that tapentadol IR (50 mg) and oxycodone IR (10 mg) provide equivalent analgesia, although a lower percentage of patients treated with tapentadol IR 50 mg reported nausea and/or vomiting (35% vs 59%; $P<0.001$) (**Table 7.3**). Tapentadol tablets can be given in doses of 50 mg, 75 mg, or 100 mg every 4 to 6 hours, depending on the pain intensity. The maximum daily dose is 700 mg (for the first day of treatment) and 600 mg (day 2 and after).

The analgesic activity of tapentadol is limited to the primary molecule, and no enzymes are needed to convert it to an active metabolite (as is the case with tramadol or codeine).[37] This implies fewer, if any, individual variations in its action compared with opioids whose pharmacology is influenced by polymorphic enzymes. No dosage adjustment is needed in mild or moderate renal impairment. Little information exists regarding tapentadol dosing in opioid-dependent patients. Data taken from a 90-day safety trial in which some patients had been taking opioids prior to enrollment suggest that tapentadol doses of 100 mg every 4 hours may be appropriate.[37]

Like other opioid agonists, tapentadol is associated with nausea, vomiting, respiratory depression, and sedation; in addition, it may in rare situations precipitate serotonin syndrome. Serotonin syndrome is characterized by mental-status changes (eg, agitation, hallucinations, hyperreflexia) and autonomic instability (eg, tachycardia, labile blood pressure, hyperthermia). The risk of serotonin syndrome is increased with concomitant administration of selective serotonin reuptake inhibitors (SSRIs), SNRIs, and monoamine oxidase inhibitors (MAOIs).[37] Tapentadol has an abuse potential similar to hydromorphone and is subject to criminal diversion. After 90 days of continuous administration, abrupt discontinuation of tapentadol was associated

TABLE 7.3 — Percentages of Patients Experiencing Nausea and Vomiting in Randomized, Double-Blind, Placebo-Controlled Studies of Tapentadol IR

	Adverse Event	Placebo	Tapentadol IR			Oxycodone HCl IR (10 or 15 mg)
			50 mg	75 mg	100 mg	
Phase 3 Study						
Bunionectomy	Nausea	13	35	38	49	67
	Vomiting	3	18	21	32	42
	Nausea and/or vomiting	—	—	41[a]	53[b]	70
Bunionectomy						
	Nausea	17	34	46	—	57
	Vomiting	0	12	28	—	26
	Nausea and/or vomiting	—	35[c]	51[d]	—	59
End-stage joint disease	Nausea	5	18	21	—	41
	Vomiting	4	7	14	—	34
	Nausea and/or vomiting	—	22[c]	30[c]	—	57

[a] $P=0.01$ not vs oxycodone HCL IR 10 mg.
[b] $P=0.007$ vs oxycodone HCl IR 10 mg.
[c] $P<0.001$ vs oxycodone HCl IR 10 mg.
[d] $P=0.057$ vs oxycodone HCl IR 10 mg.

Daniels SE, et al. *Curr Med Res Opin*. 2009;25:765-776.

7

with mild-to-moderate withdrawal symptoms in 17% of patients.[37]

■ Methadone (Dolophine)

Methadone is a synthetic phenylpropylamide-type opioid agonist with approximately 1.5 to 2 times the potency of morphine. Following oral administration, methadone is well absorbed, having a bioavailability that approaches 80%.[2-4] It also has a large volume of distribution and a prolonged, yet variable (12 to 120 hours), plasma elimination half-life.[2,3] Oral dosing of methadone is complicated and overdosage and underdosage are common. Despite its prolonged elimination half-life, methadone's redistribution half-life and duration of effect are limited. Initial oral doses provide up to 6 hours of analgesia but as drug accumulates in tissue, analgesic duration and risk of overdosing may increase substantially.[4] In addition to its activity at opioid receptors, methadone appears to provide additional analgesic effects via interactions with NMDA and α-adrenergic receptors.[2,26]

Methadone is recommended for patients suffering postsurgical nerve injuries and neuropathic pain, as well as individuals who are highly opioid dependent or opioid hyperalgesic.[2,16,38,39] Orally administered methadone is metabolized by the hepatic microsomal enzyme system undergoing *N*-demethylation or deamination into inactive compounds.[2] Methadone is available as an oral elixir or oral tablets.

■ Tramadol (Ultram)

Tramadol is a weak μ-receptor opioid agonist with equivalent potency to codeine. Tramadol also has α-adrenergic analgesic effects that complement the opioid-mediated effect.[2,4,5,40,41] It is not recommended for severe acute pain but is used for mild-to-moderate discomfort following minor surgery. In acute pain settings, doses of tramadol should not exceed 300 mg/day, and it should not be prescribed to patients taking MAOIs as it may induce psychotic behavior.[2,40,41] Tramadol also inhibits serotonin reuptake and can cause serotonin syndrome.[2,40] Tramadol is metabolized by CYP2D6 into an active metabolite that has 200 times greater μ-receptor affinity and has five times greater potency than the parent compound.[3,31] As with codeine, approximately 20% of individuals have CYP2D6 enzyme polymorphisms that result in poor metabolism. These patients cannot form the active metabolite and are at increased risk for analgesic failure.[2,40,41]

■ Meperidine (Demerol)

Meperidine is a weak synthetic opioid agonist with an oral potency equivalent to one tenth that of morphine.[2-4] Its analgesic onset is slightly more rapid than morphine, but its duration of effect is only two thirds as long. Meperidine was initially developed as an anticholinergic and provides a smooth muscle-relaxing effect.[2,5,26,42] Oral doses exceeding 1 g/day or administration to patients with renal failure may result in neurotoxicity secondary to the accumulation of its neurotoxic metabolite, normeperidine.[2,26] In addition, meperidine elevates serotonin levels and can precipitate a serotonergic crisis when coadministered with drugs that elevate serotonin, such as MAOIs.[42] Meperidine tablets are increasingly restricted in hospital settings and should never be considered for chronic pain management.[42,43]

■ Fentanyl (Sublimaze)

Fentanyl is a synthetic, μ-specific opioid agonist related to meperidine.[2] Oral doses are potent (25 to 40 times greater than morphine), have a rapid onset, and 60- to 90-minute duration of effect. Fentanyl's side effect profile is lower than that observed with morphine, although dose-dependent nausea, sedation, and pruritus are commonly observed. Major adverse effects include rapid and profound respiratory depression and severe nausea and vomiting. Fentanyl is available as a transdermal patch and a transmucosal oral lozenge (Actiq oralet).[1,2] Approximately 30% of analgesic effect provided by the oral lozenge is via direct absorption through the oral mucosa. None of these preparations are approved for postsurgical pain management. Fentanyl oralet may be considered for patients with breakthrough pain who cannot tolerate oral opioid tablets.

■ Codeine

Codeine is a naturally occurring opiate-derived analgesic that is one fourth to one third as potent as morphine.[2,3] Oral doses of codeine are used primarily in patients recovering from dental and ear, nose, and throat (ENT) surgery. Its analgesic efficacy is inferior to that of oxycodone, while its side effect profile, particularly nausea and vomiting, is higher.[2,4,26] Codeine is a prodrug that must be metabolized to morphine by CYP2D6 to achieve analgesic effect.[1,2,13,26] This enzyme is polymorphic; most patients are rapid or intermediate metabolizers.[2,26] Approximately 20% of individuals are poor metabolizers who experience a high incidence of analgesic failure. Others who are extensive metabolizers are at increased risk for morphine-related adverse effects, including excessive sedation and respiratory depression. Codeine is available as an oral tablet compounded with acetaminophen (Tylenol #3) that offers no analgesic advantages over compounded oxycodone or hydrocodone.

■ Buprenorphine (Subutex, Suboxone, BuTrans)

Buprenorphine is a partial agonist-type opioid that has been widely used as an IV analgesic in the European Union.[2,26,44] Buprenorphine has a high μ-receptor affinity and occupation rate, and for this reason, greater than normal doses of agonists or antagonists are required to displace it and reverse its effects.

A sublingual formulation of buprenorphine (Subutex) and buprenorphine plus naloxone (Suboxone) are increasingly used as maintenance therapy for opioid-dependent patients and for pain management.[45] Patients presenting for surgery should continue taking these formulations during the perioperative period as both can provide effective pain control.

Additional pain control can be provided with a fentanyl infusion, fentanyl lozenge, regional techniques, and the use of nonopioid analgesics. Alternatively, patients treated with buprenorphine can be converted to 30 mg to 40 mg of methadone/day 1 week prior to surgery to prevent withdrawal and to avoid antagonism of standard opioid analgesics.[45]

A new transdermal buprenorphine formulation (BuTrans) that provides a 7-day duration of effect is available for chronic mild-to-moderate pain.[46] Currently, transdermal buprenorphine is not approved for surgical pain management, and whether it should be continued perioperatively has not been determined.

A list of opioid analgesics commonly used for postsurgical pain management and recommendations for dose conversion are outlined in **Table 7.4**.

Future Directions With Oral and Parenteral Opioids for Postsurgical Pain

In the near future, improved and more selective opioid analgesics may be developed that better suit individual patient needs[47]:

- Rapidly disintegrating and readily absorbed lingual and buccal preparations avoid gastric absorption and first-pass hepatic metabolism and offer advantages of convenience and rapid analgesic onset. While originally developed for breakthrough chronic pain, these routes of delivery may become available for acute pain management. Nasal- and pulmonary-delivered opioid preparations offer similar advantages as well as convenience and may displace the need for IV dosing and possibly IV-PCA in patients who remain on an NPO regimen.
- Improved formulations may provide analgesic potentiation and opioid-sparing effects by compounding opioids with either α_2 agonists

TABLE 7.4 — Dosing Guidelines for Oral and Parenteral Opioids

Opioid	Route	Dose (mg)	Onset	Duration	Comments
Morphine	PO	30 (15-45)	45 min	4-5 hr	Poor oral effect, active metabolite
Morphine	IV	10 (5-15)	10 min	3.5-4 hr	Histamine release
Meperidine	PO	200 (1-300)	45 min	3.5 hr	Toxic metabolite
Meperidine	IV	100 (75-125)	10 min	3 hr	Useful for visceral pain
Hydrocodone	PO	15 (7.5-15)	35 min	4-6 hr	Similar to oxycodone
Oxycodone	PO	10 (5-15)	30 min	4-6 hr	Good oral analgesic
Codeine	PO	50 (30-70)	45 min	3.5 hr	High side effect profile
Methadone	PO	10 (7.5-15)	10-20 min	6-8 hr	Prolonged elimination
Methadone	IV	1.5-7.5 (5-10)	5-10 min	6-8 hr	Difficult to titrate
Hydromorphone	PO	15 (7.5-15)	35 min	3.5-4 hr	Well tolerated
Hydromorphone	IV	2 (1-3)	10-15 min	3.5-4 hr	Useful for severe pain
Oxymorphone	PO	10 (5-15)	30 min	5-6 hr	Poor oral bioavailability
Oxymorphone	IV	1 (0.5-2)	5-10 min	4 hr	Useful for severe pain
Fentanyl	PO (Oralet)	200-1200 mcg	5-10 min	120 min	Rapid onset
Fentanyl	IV	100-150 mcg	3-5 min	30-60 min	Very rapid onset
Tramadol	PO	100 (1-200)	40 min	4-6 hr	For mild-to-moderate pain
Tapentadol	PO	75 (50-100)	32 min	4-6 hr	Dual-acting, equipotent to oxycodone 10 mg

Values listed represent approximations based on single-dose calculations. According to this conversion scheme, IV morphine is assigned a potency of "1" while oral morphine is considered 0.3 due to its poor bioavailability and higher dose requirement. Methadone values represent single-dose effects; accumulation of drug and duration of action will increase with continued dosing.

To calculate oral-to-oral dose conversions, determine the prior 24-hour opioid dose (both scheduled and rescue doses), then utilize opioids according to the PO equianalgesic dose and potency listed above. Utilize the following proportion: "Potency of current opioid" over "24-hour dose of current opioid", multiplied by "potency of new opioid" over "X". Solve for X by cross multiplication. X equals the 24-hour dose of the new opioid. Divide the 24-hour dose and administer in increments according to the duration of action of the new drug.

For patient safety, consider using ½ to ⅓ less drug than the amount calculated. To calculate approximate IV-to-PO equianalgesic dose, utilize the table and multiply the potency of the currently used IV opioid by the prior 24-hour dose in mg. Divide this value by the potency of the PO opioid to which the patient will be converted. This value is administered in divided doses based on the duration of the PO opioid. To provide greater patient safety, divide this calculated dose by ⅓ to ½ and gauge its effectiveness. Subsequent dosing may be increased or decreased as necessary.

Adapted from Anderson R, et al. *J Pain Symptom Manage*. 2001;21(5):397-406; Sinatra RS, et al, eds. *Acute Pain Management*. London, UK: Cambridge University Press; 2009:188-203.

7

(tapentadol-like drugs) and α_2-δ antagonists such as pregabalin.

- Opioids with a lower risk of diversion and abuse. Opioids formulated in crush-resistant, water-insoluble tablets may provide a lower risk for diversion, adulteration, and abuse (snorting, injecting). Tablets containing mixtures of an agonist plus an antagonist that is released if the tablet is adulterated are also being studied.

REFERENCES

1. Sinatra RS, Torres J, Bustos AM. Pain management after major orthopaedic surgery: current strategies and new concepts. *J Am Acad Orthop Surg*. 2002;10(2):117-129.
2. Gutstein HB, Akil H. Opioid analgesics. In: Hardman JG, Limbird LE, Gilman AG, eds. *Goodman and Gilman's The Pharmacological Basis of Therapeutics*. 10th ed. New York, NY: McGraw-Hill; 2002:569-619.
3. Pasero C, Portenoy RK, McCaffery M. Opioid analgesics. In: McCaffery M, Pasero C. *Pain Clinical Manual*. St. Louis, MO: Mosby, Inc; 1999:161-299.
4. Way WL, Fields HL, Schumaker MA. Opioid analgesics. In: Katsung BG, ed. *Basic and Clinical Pharmacology*. 9th ed. New York, NY: Lange Medical Books/McGraw-Hill; 2004.
5. Fine PG, Portenoy RK. *A Clinical Guide to Opioid Analgesia*. Minneapolis, MN: McGraw-Hill Healthcare Information; 2004.
6. Sinatra R. Opioid analgesics in primary care: challenges and new advances in the management of noncancer pain. *J Am Board Fam Med*. 2006;19(2):165-177.
7. Yeh SY, Gorodetzky CW, Krebs HA. Isolation and identification of morphine 3-and 6-glucuronides, morphine 3,6-diglucuronide, morphine 3-ethereal sulfate, normorphine, and normorphine 6-glucuronide as morphine metabolites in humans. *J Pharm Sci*. 1977;66(9):1288-1293.
8. Inturrisi CE, Portenoy R, Stillman M, Colburn W, Foley K. Hydromorphone bioavailability and pharmacokinetic-pharmacodynamic (PK-PD) relationships. *Clin Pharmacol Ther*. 1988;43:162-169.
9. Keeri-Szanto M. Anaesthesia time/dose curves IX: the use of hydromorphone in surgical anaesthesia and postoperative pain relief in comparison to morphine. *Can Anaesth Soc J*. 1976; 23(6):587-595.
10. Babul N, Darke AC, Hagen N. Hydromorphone metabolite accumulation in renal failure. *J Pain Symptom Manage*. 1995; 10(3):184-186.
11. Sinatra RS, Harrison DM, Hyde N. Oxymorphone revisited. In: Katz R, ed. *Essays in Anesthesiology*. 1988;8:208-215.
12. Sinatra RS, Harrison DM. A comparison of oxymorphone and fentanyl as narcotic supplements in general anesthesia. *J Clin Anesth*. 1989;1(4):253-258.

13. Sinatra RS, Lodge K, Sibert K, et al. A comparison of morphine, meperidine, and oxymorphone as utilized in patient-controlled analgesia following cesarean delivery. *Anesthesiology.* 1989;70(4):585-590.

14. Sinatra RS. Treatment guidelines and unpublished observations. Yale University Pain Management Service; 2007.

15. Latta KS, Ginsberg B, Barkin RL. Meperidine: a critical review. *Am J Ther*. 2002;9(1):53-68.

16. Alford DP, Compton P, Samet JH. Acute pain management for patients receiving maintenance methadone or buprenorphine therapy. *Ann Intern Med.* 2006;144(2):127-134.

17. Gourlay GK, Willis RJ, Wilson PR. Postoperative pain control with methadone: influence of supplementary methadone doses and blood concentration—response relationships. *Anesthesiology*. 1984;61(1):19-26.

18. Chui PT, Gin T. A double-blind randomised trial comparing postoperative analgesia after perioperative loading doses of methadone or morphine. *Anaesth Intensive Care.* 1992;20(1):46-51.

19. Shir Y, Rosen G, Zeldin A, Davidson EM. Methadone is safe for treating hospitalized patients with severe pain. *Can J Anaesth.* 2001;48(11):1109-1113.

20. Eap CB, Buclin T, Baumann P. Interindividual variability of the clinical pharmacokinetics of methadone: implications for the treatment of opioid dependence. *Clin Pharmacokinet.* 2002;41(14):1153-1193.

21. Fishman SM, Wilsey B, Mahajan G, Molina P. Methadone reincarnated: novel clinical applications with related concerns. *Pain Med.* 2002;3(4):339-348.

22. Wedam EF, Bigelow GE, Johnson RE, Nuzzo PA, Haigney MC. QT-interval effects of methadone, levomethadyl, and buprenorphine in a randomized trial. *Arch Intern Med.* 2007; 167(22):2469-2475.

23. Peng PW, Sandler AN. A review of the use of fentanyl analgesia in the management of acute pain in adults. *Anesthesiology.* 1999;90(2):576-599.

24. Vadlivelu N, Mitra S, Nrayan D. Recent advances in postoperative pain mangement. *Yale J Biol Med.* 2010;83(1):11-25.

25. Senagore AJ, Delaney CP, Mekhail N, Dugan A, Fazio VW. Randomized clinical trial comparing epidural anaesthesia and patient-controlled analgesia after laparoscopic segmental colectomy. *Br J Surg*. 2004;90(10):1195-1199.

26. Sinatra RS. Oral and parenteral opioids. In: Sinatra RS, Viscusi G, de Leon-Cassasola O, Ginsberg B. *Acute Pain Management*. London, England: Cambridge Press; 2009.

27. McCormack JP, Warriner CB, Levine M, Glick N. A comparison of regularly dosed oral morphine and on-demand intramuscular morphine in the treatment of postsurgical pain. *Can J Anaesth*. 1993;40(9):819-824.

28. Marco CA, Plewa MC, Buderer N, Black C, Roberts A. Comparison of oxycodone and hydrocodone for the treatment of acute pain associated with fractures: a double-blind, randomized, controlled trial. *Acad Emerg Med*. 2005;12(4):282-288.

29. Ross FB, Smith MT. The intrinsic antinociceptive effects of oxycodone appear to be kappa-opioid receptor mediated. *Pain*. 1997;73(2):151-157.

30. Palangio M, Wideman GL, Keffer M, et al. Combination hydrocodone and ibuprofen versus combination oxycodone and acetaminophen in the treatment of postoperative obstetric or gynecologic pain. *Clin Ther*. 2000;22(5):600-612.

31. Singla N, Pong A, Newman K; MD-10 Study Group. Combination oxycodone 5 mg/ibuprofen 400 mg for the treatment of pain after abdominal or pelvic surgery in women: a randomized, double-blind, placebo- and active-controlled parallel-group study. *Clin Ther*. 2005;27(1):45-57.

32. Ginsberg B, Sinatra RS, Adler LJ, et al. Conversion to oral controlled-release oxycodone from intravenous opioid analgesic in the postoperative setting. *Pain Med*. 2003;4(1):31-38.

33. Mahler DL, Forrest WH Jr. Relative analgesic potencies of morphine and hydromorphone in postoperative pain. *Anesthesiology*. 1975;42(5):602-607.

34. Ritschel WA, Parab PV, Denson DD, Coyle DE, Gregg RV. Absolute bioavailability of hydromorphone after peroral and rectal administration in humans: saliva/plasma ratio and clinical effects. *J Clin Pharmacol*. 1987;27(9):647-653.

35. Opana ER (oxymorphone hydrochloride) extended-release tablets [package insert]. Chadds Ford, PA: Endo Pharmaceuticals Inc; September 2010.

36. Aqua K, Gimbel JS, Singla N, Ma T, Ahdieh H, Kerwin R. Efficacy and tolerability of oxymorphone immediate release for acute postoperative pain after abdominal surgery: a randomized, double-blind, active- and placebo-controlled, parallel-group trial. *Clin Ther*. 2007;29(6):1000-1012.

37. Nucynta (tapentadol) immediate-release oral tablets [package insert]. Princeton, NJ: Ortho-McNeil Pharmaceuticals; 2010.

38. Hartrick C, Van Hove I, Stegmann JU, Oh C, Upmalis D. Efficacy and tolerability of tapentadol immediate release and oxycodone HCl immediate release in patients awaiting primary joint replacement surgery for end-stage joint disease: a 10-day, phase III, randomized, double-blind, active- and placebo-controlled study. *Clin Ther*. 2009;31(2):260-271.

39. Rowbotham MC, Twilling L, Davies PS, Reisner L, Taylor K, Mohr D. Oral opioid therapy for chronic peripheral and central neuropathic pain. *N Engl J Med*. 2003;348(13):1223-1232.

40. Sinatra RS, Sramcik J. Tramadol: its use in pain management. *Anesthesiol Clin North America*. 1998;2:53-69.

41. Dayer P, Desmeules J, Collart L. [Pharmacology of tramadol]. *Drugs*. 1997;53(suppl 2):18-24. French.

42. Latta KS, Ginsberg B, Barkin RL. Meperidine: a critical review. *Am J Ther*. 2002;9(1):53-68.

43. Raymo LL, Camejo M, Fudin J. Eradicating analgesic use of meperidine in a hospital. *Am J Health Syst Pharm*. 2007;64 (11):1148, 1150, 1152.

44. Abrahamsson J, Niemand D, Olsson AK, Törnebrandt K. [Buprenorphine (Temgesic) as a peroperative analgesic. A multicenter study]. *Anaesthesist*. 1983;32(2):75-79. German.

45. Heit HA, Gourlay DL. Buprenorphine: new tricks with an old molecule for pain management. *Clin J Pain*. 2008;24(2):93-97.

46. James IG, O'Brien CM, McDonald CJ. A randomized, double-blind, double-dummy comparison of the efficacy and tolerability of low-dose transdermal buprenorphine (BuTrans seven-day patches) with buprenorphine sublingual tablets (Temgesic) in patients with osteoarthritis pain. *J Pain Symptom Manage*. 2010;40(2):266-278.

47. National Institutes of Health. *The NIH Guide: New Directions in Pain Research I*. Washington, DC: US Government Printing Office; 1998.

8

NSAIDs and COX-2 Inhibitors

by Raymond S. Sinatra, MD, PhD

Introduction

Nonsteroidal anti-inflammatory drugs (NSAIDs) represent a large and varied class of peripherally acting analgesics that are among the most widely used pain medications worldwide. The class is well known to patients and surgeons alike, with over 70 million prescription-strength doses written every year and a large number of over-the-counter formulations readily available for use.[1,2]

8

In the perioperative setting, NSAIDs play a key role in multimodal analgesia and are prescribed as alternatives or adjuncts to opioid-based analgesia. NSAIDs possess analgesic and anti-inflammatory, as well as antipyretic, properties and have proven efficacy in the treatment of headache, osteoarthritis, and postsurgical pain. In addition to oral tablets and transdermal preparations, two IV-administered NSAIDs, ketorolac (Toradol) and ibuprofen (Caldolor), have been approved for surgical pain management in the United States.[3,4]

Site and Mechanism of Activity

The primary mechanism by which NSAIDs exert their analgesic effects is by inhibition of arachidonic acid–COX pathways.[1,2,5-7] Two distinct pathways mediated by cyclooxygenase isoforms, COX-1 and COX-2, have been identified.[5,6] Cyclooxygenase-1 is the normally expressed, homeostatic isoform that promotes platelet aggregation, renal blood flow, and gastric protection. In contrast, COX-2 is minimally expressed in normal settings but is markedly upregulated following trauma or surgery[5] (**Figure 8.1**). Following tissue injury, arachidonic acid is released from damaged cell membranes and converted by COX-2 into prostaglandin E_2 (PGE_2). PGE_2 plays a critical role in nociceptor activation and initiation of the inflammatory cascade.[1,2,5]

By inhibiting COX-2 and reducing PGE_2 synthesis, NSAIDs decrease inflammatory hyperalgesia and allodynia (pain associated with innocuous stimulation).[1,5] NSAIDs also block the recruitment of leukocytes and monocytes and production of cytokines and other leukocyte-derived inflammatory mediators.[1,2,6,7] Some NSAIDs are able to cross the blood-brain barrier, where they limit PGE_2 synthesis in sensitized neurons and glial cells.[8] In this manner, NSAIDs reduce local inflammation and can prevent both peripheral and central sensitization.

No analgesic class is without adverse effects, and NSAIDs are no exception. Common adverse effects of nonselective NSAIDs are related to their inhibition of homeostatic PGs and the resulting increase in risks of GI bleeding, platelet dysfunction, and renal failure.[1,5,9] NSAIDs are contraindicated for the treatment of perioperative pain in the setting of coronary artery bypass graft (CABG) surgery, and caution is required in patients with a variety of common conditions, including asthma, hypertension, renal insufficiency, preexisting ulcer disease, and CHF, among others.[1,2,9,10]

Prior to administration, clinicians must weigh potential advantages of NSAIDs, including reductions in opioid dose, vs their impact on surgical hemostasis and other aspects of patient safety. Not all NSAIDs are alike, therefore agent-specific toxicity, black box warnings, COX-1 specificity, cost, and route of administration must also be considered.[1,10,11]

FIGURE 8.1 — Mechanism of Action of NSAIDs and Coxibs

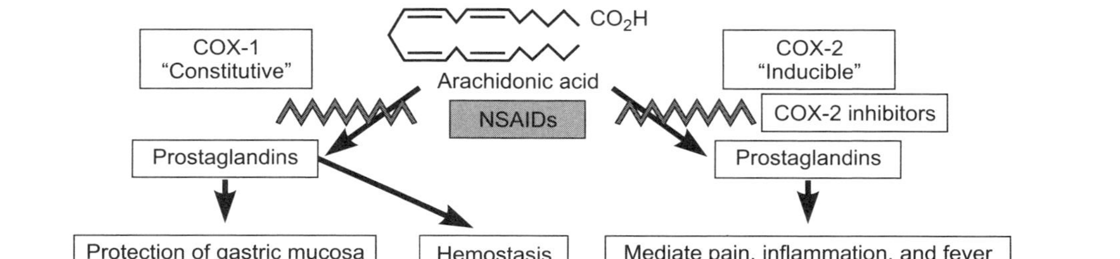

Two forms of cyclooxygenase, COX-1 and COX-2, have been identified. COX-1 is primarily responsible for the synthesis of constitutive or protective PGEs, which mediate the normal function of platelets, the kidneys, and the GI tract. The COX-2 isoform is induced following tissue injury and is primarily responsible for the synthesis of PGEs that initiate and maintain pain and inflammation. By inhibiting COX-1, NSAIDs diminish levels of PGE, which may result in GI ulceration, impaired wound-site hemostasis, and renal dysfunction. The analgesic effects of NSAIDs are related to their inhibition of COX-2 and subsequent reduction in PGEs that cause pain inflammation and fever. Studies of selective COX-2 inhibitors have revealed an enhanced risk for CV events.

Modified from Vane JR, Botting RM. *Inflamm Res*. 1995;44(1):1-10.

Injectable Ketorolac

Ketorolac tromethamine (Toradol) was the first injectable NSAID approved for use by the FDA, and has been widely prescribed for surgical pain management for >20 years. It is indicated for the short-term (≤5 days) management of moderate-to-moderately severe postsurgical pain.[3] A number of studies have evaluated the efficacy of IV ketorolac in postsurgical settings, noting significant reductions in pain, opioid-sparing effects, and facilitation of recovery.[12-14] Ketorolac administered alone in doses of 30 mg to 60 mg is as potent as 10 mg of morphine and is particularly useful in managing surgical and posttraumatic musculoskeletal pain and visceral pain.[14] When employed as a multimodal analgesic, a 30-mg loading dose of ketorolac, followed by 15-mg to 30-mg doses every 6 hours, provides useful augmentation of opioid-based analgesia or neural blockade.[1,2] Unlike opioids, it is not associated with excessive sedation, cognitive dysfunction, or respiratory depression.

In contrast to many other NSAIDs, ketorolac is an extreme outlier in terms of its inhibitory effect on COX-1 relative to COX-2[5] (**Figure 8.2**). This finding has important safety-related implications for perioperative use, since the negative effect of NSAIDs on renal function, GI mucosal integrity, and platelet function is the direct result of COX-1 inhibition.[1,2,5,15] Platelet dysfunction associated with ketorolac can increase the risk for postsurgical hematomas, wound-site bleeding, and life-threatening occult bleeding.[5,10] For this reason, ketorolac has been withdrawn from the European market. In the United States, IV ketorolac is contraindicated in patients who have a history of GI bleeding or who are at risk for major postsurgical bleeding. As such, the prescribing information for IV ketorolac contains a black box warning against its use as a prophylactic analgesic prior to any form of major surgery.[3] In an effort to reduce dose-dependent COX-1 interactions, we recommend that postsurgical doses

FIGURE 8.2 — Inhibition of COX-2 Relative to COX-1

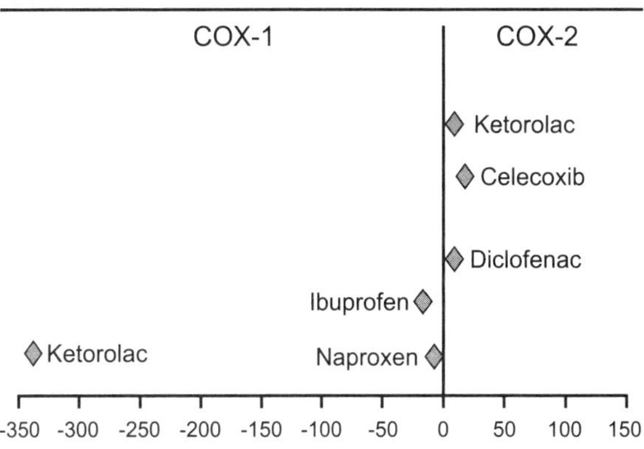

Currently, there are two injectable NSAIDs available for use in the United States: ibuprofen injection (Caldolor) and ketorolac (Toradol). While both are nonselective NSAIDs, they differ in their degree of inhibition of COX-2 relative to COX-1. Ibuprofen inhibits COX-1 2.5 times more than COX-2, whereas ketorolac inhibits COX-1 >300 times more than COX-2.

Adapted from Warner TD, et al. *Proc Natl Acad Sci U S A*. 1999; 96(13):7563-7568.

8

of ketorolac be reduced to 7.5 mg to 10 mg every 6 hours and given for no longer than 48 hours as part of a multimodal approach to surgical pain.

Ibuprofen Injection (Caldolor)

An injectable formulation of ibuprofen (Caldolor) was approved for use in the United States in June 2009, and it is indicated for management of mild-to-moderate pain by itself, and for management of moderate-to-severe pain as an adjunct to opioid analgesics.[4] Similar to oral ibuprofen, the IV formulation inhibits both COX-1 and COX-2. When compared with IV ketorolac, the ibuprofen injection has a more "balanced" affinity for the COX isoenzymes (**Figure 8.2**). Lower selectivity for COX-1 may translate into reduced risk of platelet dysfunction and GI ulceration.[4,10,11,15]

Recommended dosing guidelines for ibuprofen injection are 800 mg every 6 hours, with a maximum 24-hour dose of 3200 mg. Elderly and low-weight patients (>50 kg) may experience effective pain control with 400-mg doses. The drug is supplied in vials containing either 400 mg or 800 mg of ibuprofen in 4 mL to 8 mL of clear solution. Unlike ketorolac, the drug should never be given as a rapid IV bolus. Instead, the contents of each vial should be diluted in 250-mL bags of sterile saline or lactated Ringer's, and infused over a period of 7 to 15 minutes.[4] By following these dosing recommendations, maximal plasma concentrations (C_{max}) achieved with the 800-mg ibuprofen injection are double that observed with 800 mg of oral ibuprofen, and time to C_{max} is considerably more rapid. These pharmacokinetic differences increase drug concentrations at the site of tissue injury and underscore rapid onset and high analgesic efficacy of the ibuprofen injection.

In a randomized, double-blind, placebo-controlled trial, the safety and efficacy of ibuprofen injection was evaluated in 319 patients undergoing abdominal hysterectomy.[16] Injectable ibuprofen 800 mg given at wound closure and every 6 hours for up to 5 days was associated with significant reductions in pain with movement (14% reduction at 24 hours vs placebo; $P=0.010$) and a 19% reduction in 24-hour morphine requirements ($P\leq0.001$). When compared with patients treated with placebo, there was no difference in treatment-emergent adverse events, including wound-site bleeding, reduced hematocrit, and renal toxicity.

Singla and colleagues evaluated the safety and efficacy of an intravenous ibuprofen administered preemptively as a multimodal analgesic.[17] One hundred and eighty-five patients undergoing major orthopedic surgery received either 800 mg IV ibuprofen or placebo prior to surgical incision, then every 6 hours for up to

5 days following surgery. Patients receiving ibuprofen injection required 31% less PCA morphine over the first 24 hours ($P \leq 0.001$). They also experienced reductions in pain at rest (32% vs placebo; $P<0.001$) and with movement (26% vs placebo; $P<0.001$) (**Figure 8.3**). These data indicate that ibuprofen injection offers greater analgesic efficacy when administered preoperatively. Preincisional administration did not reduce overall patient safety, as there were no differences in surgical bleeding, renal toxicity, or other adverse events between the study groups.

Ibuprofen injections are well tolerated by high-risk patients. No renal, GI, or hemostatic abnormalities were noted in debilitated burn-injured patients receiving multiple doses of ibuprofen injection for control of fever.[4] Like other NSAIDs, ibuprofen injection should

8

FIGURE 8.3 — Pain Assessed With Movement

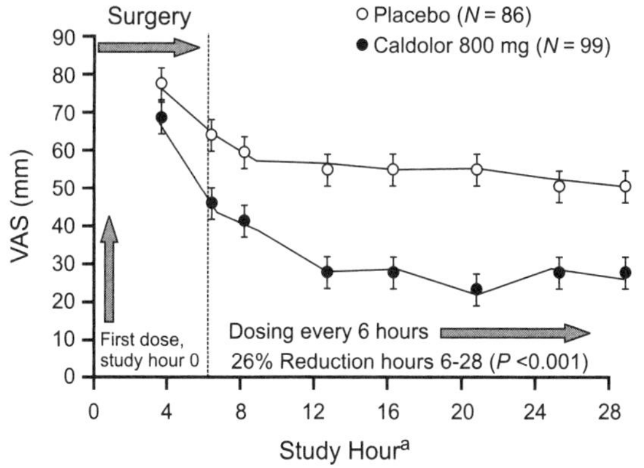

Patients treated with presurgical ibuprofen injection (800 mg), followed by repeated doses every 6 hours, awoke in less pain and remained in less pain throughout the postoperative period. Patients experienced a 26% reduction in pain intensity scores when pain was assessed with movement.

[a] Statistical significance was demonstrated at each assessment point.

Adapted from Singla N, et al. *Pain Med.* 2010;11(8):1284-1293.

be withheld in patients with active GI ulcers or prerenal azotemia, as well as patients with anticipated or ongoing surgical-site bleeding, and in those recovering from CABG surgery.[4]

COX-2 Inhibitors

Research and development of the COX-2 inhibitors was driven by the need to improve GI safety while maintaining analgesic efficacy.[1,5,11] In this regard, 60% of patients taking nonselective NSAIDs report GI tract adverse effects. COX-2 inhibitors, or coxibs, are a subclass of NSAIDs that are relatively more specific for the COX-2 enzyme isoform compared with COX-1. Selective inhibition of COX-2 provides powerful anti-inflammatory and antinociceptive effects without compromising the constitutive benefits of COX-1.[1,5,10,11] Following long-term coxib administration, the incidence of gastric ulcer is similar to that observed with placebo, and significantly lower than that observed with nonselective NSAIDs.[5,10] Despite this increase in safety, the COX-2 inhibitors should not be given to patients with active bleeding ulcers. Current guidelines suggest pairing a COX-2 inhibitor with a proton pump inhibitor in patients with a prior history of GI bleeding.[1,2] An additional clinical benefit of coxibs is that they have no effect on platelet function. They do not prolong the bleeding time and do not increase risks of wound-site or occult bleeding.[1,5,10,11]

The first COX-2 inhibitor approved by the FDA in 1998 was celecoxib (Celebrex). Following the withdrawal of rofecoxib (Vioxx) and valdecoxib (Bextra), celecoxib is the only COX-2 inhibitor currently available for acute pain management. The analgesic effectiveness of oral celecoxib has been confirmed and its hemostatic safety demonstrated in several surgical models.[1,2,11,18] Gimbel and colleagues[18] reported that celecoxib 200 mg provided a similar onset and overall quality of analgesia as that observed with hydrocodone 10 mg/acetaminophen 1000 mg in patients recovering from orthopedic surgery. Celecoxib was not associated with increased blood loss, and patients benefited from a lower incidence of GI adverse events.

Celecoxib is well suited for preemptive or preincisional dosing as it is not associated with impaired platelet function or prolongation of the bleeding time. Recommended dosing is 200 mg to 400 mg oral celecoxib with a small sip of water given 2 hours prior to induction of anesthesia. Thereafter, depending on patient age, weight, and comorbidity, doses of 100 mg to 200 mg can be administered every 12 hours for 5 days or longer.[19]

The FDA has mandated a black-box warning for celecoxib with regard to risks of cardiovascular and cerebrovascular thrombosis with long-term use.[19] Because of these risks, administration of celecoxib fell out of favor for several years. More recently, the efficacy and short-term safety benefits of celecoxib have been reconsidered by surgeons and anesthesiologists who are increasingly utilizing the drug for perioperative pain management.[1,2,10] To minimize cardiovascular complications, do not administer celecoxib in CABG surgery or in patients at high risk for cardiovascular and cerebrovascular thromboses.[19] Since COX-2 also has a renal protective effect and controls renin release in hypovolemic patients, celecoxib (as well as NSAIDs) is also contraindicated in prerenal azotemia.[19]

Optimizing NSAID Benefits While Reducing Risks

One criticism of analgesic regimens that employ NSAIDs or COX-2 selective inhibitors has been an inability to consistently correlate reductions in opioid consumption and improved pain control with measurable improvements in clinical outcomes and patient functionality.[1,2,10,11] Most trials have been underpowered, single-dose, short-term evaluations that could not reliably discern significant differences between treatment groups.[1,2] Clinical advantages have been detected when the results of many similar trials are pooled together. Marret and coworkers[20] published a meta-analysis of 22 randomized, double-blind studies that included 2307 postsurgical patients using IV-PCA morphine who were either treated or not treated with NSAIDs. Coadministration of NSAIDs significantly reduced the incidence of postsurgical nausea and vomiting by 30%, nausea alone by 12%, vomiting alone by 32%, and sedation by 29%. NSAIDs had no effect on pruritus, urinary retention, and respiratory depression. A regression analysis indicated that reductions in morphine consumption correlated positively with reductions in the incidence of nausea and vomiting (**Figure 8.4**). In a separate analysis of 52 randomized placebo-controlled trials, Elia and colleagues[21] compared postsurgical NSAIDs and coxib-based multimodal analgesia vs opioid monotherapy. Coadministration of NSAIDs was associated with a 15% to 55% decrease in opioid dose requirements, reductions in pain intensity at 24 hours, and a reduced incidence of nausea/vomiting (from 29% to 22%) and sedation (from 15.4% to 12.7%).

During movement and ambulation, increased tension at the incision site exacerbates tissue injury, resulting in a heightened inflammatory response and further sensitization of peripheral nociceptors. NSAIDs can attenuate this response, as evidenced by studies in which patients treated with either injectable ibuprofen[17] or rofecoxib[22] reported significant reductions in incident pain associated with movement. Buvanendran and colleagues[22] utilized a protocol designed to detect improvements in patient functionality following total knee arthroplastic surgery. Patients treated with perioperative doses of a COX-2–selective inhibitor reported improved relief of incident pain and benefited from significant increases in angle of knee flexion during rehabilitation. A well-powered clinical trial evaluating recovery from abdominal gynecologic surgery found that patients randomized to receive multiple perioperative doses of COX-2–selective inhibitors not only

FIGURE 8.4 — Coadministration of NSAIDs Reduces Postsurgical Opioid Adverse Events

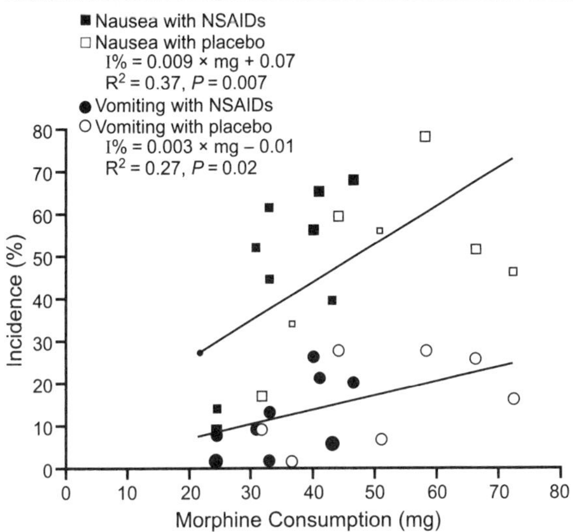

A regression analysis of nausea and vomiting from 22 postsurgical trials in which patients utilized IV-PCA morphine and were either treated or not treated with NSAIDs. Reductions in the incidence of nausea and vomiting correlated positively with reductions in morphine consumption.

Marret E, et al. *Anesthesiology*. 2005;102(6):1249-1260.

reported lower pain intensity scores and required significantly less PCA morphine, but also benefited from lower sedation scores and more rapid return of bowel function.[23] The common denominator that reduced incident pain and facilitated return of bowel function in these trials was the fact that coxibs and NSAIDs were utilized in a well-defined multimodal treatment plan; the first dose was given prior to rather than following surgery, and follow-up doses were given for extended periods of time (5 days).[17,22,23]

Despite the clear analgesic advantages offered by NSAIDs and coxibs, a large number of surgeons

8

either withhold or limit dosing in perioperative settings. Many surgeons routinely discontinue NSAIDs 5 to 10 days prior to surgery, citing risks of increased perioperative bleeding and possible inhibition of wound healing.[1,2] The withdrawal of NSAIDs prior to relatively noninvasive or low blood-loss procedures is unnecessary in most patients. Moreover, abrupt discontinuance of NSAIDs may increase preoperative discomfort and ensures that surgery is performed in a setting of increased inflammation and sensitization. If caregivers are truly concerned about potential increases in surgical bleeding, preoperative patient comfort and postsurgical safety can be maintained by discontinuing nonselective NSAIDs 3 to 5 days prior to surgery and substituting the COX-2 inhibitor celecoxib.

There is no evidence to suggest that a short-term administration of NSAIDs (24 to 36 hours) has negative effects on orthopedic surgical outcomes. Nevertheless, some orthopedic surgeons avoid NSAIDs following total joint replacement procedures as well as spinal fusion surgery, fearing that inhibition of the inflammatory response may impair bone regrowth and increase the risk of fusion or prosthetic failure. Fusion failure was reported in one retrospective trial in which relatively high doses of ketorolac were administered for prolonged periods of time.[24] We recommend that caregivers follow guidelines promoted by the ASA.[25] Unless contraindicated, NSAIDs should always be considered for postsurgical pain management, with the lowest effective dose utilized for the most appropriate duration of therapy. NSAID and coxib pharmacology and dosing guidelines are presented in **Table 8.1**.

Conclusion

Perioperative administration of injectable NSAIDs or celecoxib can attenuate peripheral inflammation and nociceptor sensitization, and should be considered a key analgesic component of the multimodal management of postsurgical pain. Parenteral NSAIDs offer

TABLE 8.1 — NSAIDs Approved for Surgical Pain Management[a]

	Celecoxib	Ibuprofen	Ketorolac
Administration	Oral	Injectable, oral	Injectable
Dose	200-400 mg load, then 100-200 mg bid	400-800 mg IV infusion over 15 min qid	15-30 mg slow IV push qid
Preoperative dosing safety	Yes	Yes	No[b]
>5-day dosing	Yes	Yes	No
COX-2 selectivity	High	Moderate	Low
COX-1 selectivity	Low	Moderate	High
GI bleeding risk	Low	Moderate	Higher
Potential CV risk	Moderate	Lower	Lower
Fever indication	No	Yes	No

[a] Per package inserts.
[b] Black box warning.

8

rapid analgesic onset and utility in patients who cannot take oral medications. A more favorable COX-1 vs COX-2 selectivity ratio, lack of restriction to preoperative dosing, and an up to 5-day dosing interval are suggestive that ibuprofen injection may offer clinical safety advantages over IV ketorolac. Several new NSAID formulations, including injectable diclofenac and intranasal ketorolac, are awaiting FDA approval for use in the United States and offer additional dosing options and versatility in postsurgical settings, as well as potential improvements in safety.

REFERENCES

1. Jahr JS, Donkor KN, Sinatra RS. Non-selective non-steroidal anti-inflammatory drugs (NSAIDs), cyclooxygenase-2 inhibitors (COX-2Is), and acetaminophen in acute perioperative pain: analgesic efficacy, opiate-sparing effects, and adverse effects. In: Sinatra RS, Leon-Cassasola OA, Viscusi ER, Ginsberg B, McQuay H, eds. *Acute Pain Management*. 2nd ed. New York, NY: Cambridge University Press; 2009:332-365.
2. Cashman JN. The mechanisms of action of NSAIDs in analgesia. *Drugs*. 1996;52(suppl 5):13-23.
3. Injectable Ketorolac (Toradol) [prescribing information]. http://www.drugs.com/pro/ketorolac-tromethamine.html. Accessed December 1, 2011.
4. Ibuprofen Injection (Caldolor) [package insert]. Nashville, TN: Cumberland Pharmaceuticals, Inc. http://caldolor.com/pdfs/Caldolor_Full_Prescribing_Information.pdf. Accessed December 1, 2011.
5. Vane JR, Botting RM. Mechanism of action of nonsteroidal anti-inflammatory drugs. *Am J Med*. 1998;104(3A):2S-8S.
6. Ong CK, Lirk P, Tan CH, Seymour RA. An evidence-based update on nonsteroidal anti-inflammatory drugs. *Clin Med Res*. 2007;5(1):19-34.
7. Sarkar S, Hobson AR, Hughes A, et al. The prostaglandin E2 receptor-1 (EP-1) mediates acid-induced visceral pain hypersensitivity in humans. *Gastroenterology*. 2003;124(1):18-25.
8. Seybold VS, Jia YP, Abrahams LG. Cyclo-oxygenase-2 contributes to central sensitization in rats with peripheral inflammation. *Pain*. 2003;105(1-2):47-55.

9. Jones R, Rubin G, Berenbaum F, Scheiman J. Gastrointestinal and cardiovascular risks of nonsteroidal anti-inflammatory drugs. *Am J Med.* 2008;121(6):464-474.

10. Pham K, Hirschberg R. Global safety of coxibs and NSAIDs. *Curr Top Med Chem.* 2005;5(5):465-473.

11. Scheiman JM. Balancing risks and benefits of cyclooxygenase-2 selective nonsteroidal anti-inflammatory drugs. *Gastroenterol Clin North Am.* 2009;38(2):305-314.

12. Wong HY, Carpenter RL, Kopacz DJ, et al. A randomized, double-blind evaluation of ketorolac tromethamine for postoperative analgesia in ambulatory surgery patients. *Anesthesiology.* 1993;78(1):6-14.

13. Cabell CA. Does ketorolac produce preemptive analgesic effects in laparoscopic ambulatory surgery patients? *AANA J.* 2000;68(4):343-349.

14. Wheatley RG. Analgesic efficacy of ketorolac. *Acta Anaesthesiol Belg.* 1996;47(3):135-142.

15. Warner TD, Giuliano F, Vojnovic I, Bukasa A, Mitchell JA, Vane JR. Nonsteroid drug selectivities for cyclo-oxygenase-1 rather than cyclo-oxygenase-2 are associated with human gastrointestinal toxicity: a full in vitro analysis. *Proc Natl Acad Sci U S A.* 1999;96(13):7563-7568.

16. Kroll PB, Meadows L, Rock A, Pavliv L. A multicenter, randomized, double-blind, placebo-controlled trial of intravenous ibuprofen (i.v.-ibuprofen) in the management of postoperative pain following abdominal hysterectomy. *Pain Pract.* 2011;11(1):23-32.

17. Singla N, Rock A, Pavliv L. A multi-center, randomized, double-blind placebo-controlled trial of intravenous-ibuprofen (IV-ibuprofen) for treatment of pain in post-operative orthopedic adult patients. *Pain Med.* 2010;11(8):1284-1293.

18. Gimbel JS, Brugger A, Zhao W, Verburg KM, Geis GS. Efficacy and tolerability of celecoxib versus hydrocodone/acetaminophen in the treatment of pain after ambulatory orthopedic surgery in adults. *Clin Ther.* 2001;23(2):228-241.

19. Celecoxib (Celebrex) [package insert]. New York: Pfizer. http://pfizer.com/files/products/uspi_celebrex.pdf. January 2011. Accessed December 1, 2011.

20. Marret E, Kurdi O, Zufferey P, Bonnet F. Effects of nonsteroidal antiinflammatory drugs on patient-controlled analgesia morphine side effects: meta-analysis of randomized controlled trials. *Anesthesiology.* 2005;102(6):1249-1260.

21. Elia N, Lysakowski C, Tramèr MR. Does multimodal analgesia with acetaminophen, nonsteroidal antiinflammatory drugs, or selective cyclooxygenase-2 inhibitors and patient-controlled analgesia morphine offer advantages over morphine alone? Meta-analyses of randomized trials. *Anesthesiology*. 2005; 103(6):1296-1304.

22. Buvanendran A, Kroin JS, Tuman KJ, et al. Effects of perioperative administration of a selective cyclooxygenase 2 inhibitor on pain management and recovery of function after knee replacement: a randomized controlled trial. *JAMA*. 2003;290(18):2411-2418.

23. Sinatra RS, Boice JA, Loeys TL, et al; Protocol 159 Study Group. Evaluation of the effect of perioperative rofecoxib treatment on pain control and clinical outcomes in patients recovering from gynecologic abdominal surgery: a randomized, double-blind, placebo-controlled clinical study. *Reg Anesth Pain Med*. 2006;31(2):134-142.

24. Glassman SD, Rose SM, Dimar JR, Puno RM, Campbell MJ, Johnson JR. The effect of postoperative nonsteroidal anti-inflammatory drug administration on spinal fusion. *Spine*. 1998;23(7):834-838.

25. Practice guidelines for acute pain management in the perioperative setting. A report by the American Society of Anesthesiologists Task Force on Pain Management, Acute Pain Section. *Anesthesiology*. 1995;82(4):1071-1081.

9

Other Analgesics and Adjuvants Used in Postsurgical Pain Management

by Raymond S. Sinatra, MD, PhD

Introduction

Analgesic adjuvants and anesthetics provide therapeutic alternatives for:

- Patients experiencing opioid intolerance
- Pain symptoms that cannot be optimally controlled with opioids alone.

9

They are often prescribed to control specific surgical- or trauma-related complaints, including:

- Skeletal muscle spasm
- Visceral muscle spasm
- Inflammation
- Neuropathic pain
- Opioid hyperalgesia.

NSAIDs, COX inhibitors, the use of local anesthetics, and acetaminophen should always be considered and, unless contraindicated, used to enhance opioid-mediated analgesia.[1] The following chapter will introduce other multimodal adjuvants that may also be considered for patients with difficult-to-manage postsurgical pain, including:

- Local anesthetics/analgesics (LAs)
- α_2-agonists
- Muscle relaxants
- Anticonvulsant analgesics
- NMDA receptor antagonists (ketamine)
- Corticosteroids
- TCAs.

Local Anesthetics/Analgesics

LAs represent a class of analgesic compounds that block conduction of noxious impulses in peripheral and spinal nerves. They are broadly classified as either "amides" or "esters" based on the nature of the linkage between the aromatic ring and the tertiary amine (**Figure 9.1**). Chemical groups attached to the aromatic ring influence the speed of onset, while groups attached to the tertiary amine influence lipid solubility and anesthetic potency.[1-3] Ester-based LAs, including procaine (Novocain), were commercially developed in the early 1900s and were widely utilized in surgical and dental practice. Amide LAs, including lidocaine (Xylocaine), were developed later in the 1960s and have since displaced esters in most clinical settings. Bupivacaine (Marcaine), an amide LA with a longer duration of action, was introduced in 1972 and, finally, EXPAREL (bupivacaine liposome injectable suspension) in 2011 that has up to a 72-hour duration of action.

In contrast to most drugs used in pain medicine, LAs are only effective when injected in the vicinity of pain fibers innervating the surgical wound site.[2,3] LAs

FIGURE 9.1 — Chemical Components of Ester- and Amide-Based Local Anesthetics

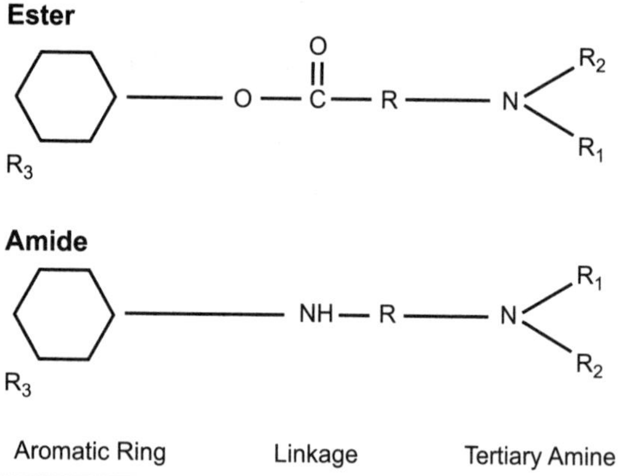

Ester

R_3 (aromatic ring) — O — C(=O) — R — N(R_2)(R_1)

Amide

R_3 (aromatic ring) — NH — R — N(R_1)(R_2)

Aromatic Ring | Linkage | Tertiary Amine

act by reversibly interfering with both the initiation and propagation of neuronal action potentials. They do this by blocking Na^+ influx through voltage-gated sodium channels in the axonal membrane.[2,3] Noxious C and Aδ fibers tend to localize at the periphery of a nerve bundle and are more vulnerable to LA blockade than the motor fibers located in the core (**Figure 9.2**). Some LAs, such as bupivacaine (Marcaine), EXPAREL (bupivacaine liposome injectable suspension), and ropivacaine (Naropin), can also differentially block the sodium channel by a process termed "frequency-

FIGURE 9.2 — Anatomic Correlates of Local Anesthetic Blockade

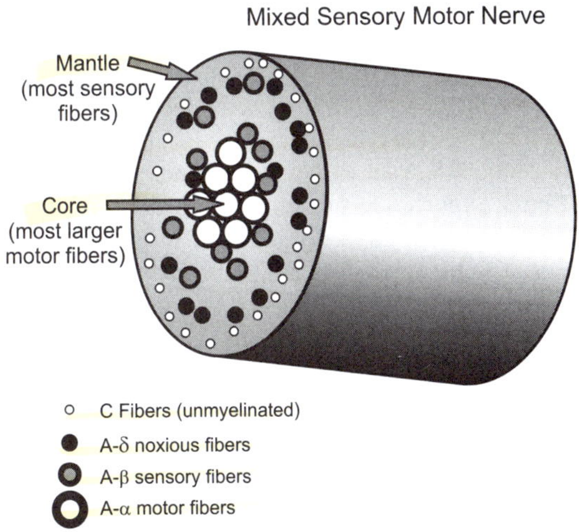

In mixed sensory nerves, noxious C fibers and Aδ fibers are generally localized to the outer regions of the nerve, *(mantle)* while larger motor and sensory fibers are localized in the center of the nerve *(core)*. Because of a concentration gradient from the site of local anesthetic deposition to the center of the nerve, the mantle fibers are first to be blocked and last to recover. As local anesthetic diffuses further into the nerve, core fibers are blocked, although they are first to recover. This orientation of fibers favors selective conduction blockade in noxious fibers and analgesic effects that outlast the duration of sensory/motor anesthesia.

dependent blockade."[2,4] By using dilute bupivacaine solutions, the surgeon can effectively block pain fibers firing most frequently, while sparing larger motor and sensory fibers. Differential blockade of various types of fiber with low to increasing concentrations of LA occurs in the following order: noxious > cold/warm > light touch > deep touch > proprioception > motor fibers.[2,4]

The ability of LAs to anesthetize specific regions of the body reduces or eliminates the need for general anesthesia and provides both painless surgery and effective postoperative analgesia. Applications include:

- Infiltration or localized injection into the wound
- Single-dose or continuous peripheral nerve blocks
- Central neural blockade.

Preincisional neural blockade decreases the incidence and severity of surgical-site hyperalgesia and may reduce the risk of developing persistent pain.[2,3] Patients experience minimal-to-no discomfort for several hours to days. Reductions in pain intensity are usually associated with significant opioid-sparing and decreased adverse events. LAs such as lidocaine, bupivacaine, and ropivacaine are available at low cost and, in ambulatory surgical settings, offer benefits of reduced PACU stay and less time needed to control postoperative pain. Inpatients can be discharged sooner with fewer complications, such as deep venous thrombosis, ileus, and pulmonary atelectasis. LAs are generally well tolerated and safe when administered properly. They reliably unbind from their sites of action, leaving no lasting effects.[3,4]

The duration and degree of neural blockade can be customized to specific surgical or patient needs by varying the concentration of drug, the volume administered, and for moderate- and shorter-acting agents, the addition of epinephrine and other adjuvants like clonidine and steroids.[5] Bolus doses of up to 20 to 40 mL of 0.25% to 0.5% bupivacaine or 0.2% to 0.5%

ropivacaine may be employed for infiltration or single-dose peripheral nerve block.[2,4] Solutions of 0.25% bupivacaine or ropivacaine 0.2% may be continuously infused perineurally via infusion pumps at 8 to 12 mL/hour for up to 72 hours.[6] Sites of perineural infusion include femoral, sciatic, and common tibial nerves for lower extremity procedures, supraclavicular and interscalene blocks for upper extremity surgery, and paravertebral block for thoracic and abdominal procedures.

LA-based analgesia has several disadvantages:

- Infiltration techniques, while generally straightforward, may lead to patchy or incomplete blockade if the surgeon uses too limited a dose or does not infiltrate all surgical planes of the wound site.
- When performing peripheral nerve block, LAs must be precisely injected into the desired nerve or plexus sheath. Injection may be complicated or contraindicated due to technical difficulties, patient noncooperation, infection, or anticoagulation concerns.
- LAs are associated with dose-dependent neuro- or cardiotoxicity. Toxicity is a primary concern following unintentional IV administration. LAs can also precipitate neuro- and cardiotoxicity when large doses are infiltrated into highly vascular tissues.[2,3]
- Some LAs, including lidocaine and chloroprocaine, are reasonably benign, but potent amides, such as bupivacaine and ropivacaine, are associated with seizures and fatal ventricular arrhythmias. Doses should not exceed 1.7 to 2 mg/kg with bupivacaine, 3 mg/kg with ropivacaine, 5 mg/kg with lidocaine, and 266 mg (20 mL, 1.3% of undiluted drug per surgical site with EXPAREL (bupivacaine liposome injectable suspension).
- The addition of epinephrine 1:200,000 decreases the rate of absorption and risk of toxicity.

- Treatment of LA toxicity depends on the agent and dose administered and the site of injection.[7] For example, symptoms such as dizziness or numb lips caused by lidocaine may resolve quickly with supportive care and oxygen. Cardiotoxicity observed with bupivacaine and ropivacaine usually requires airway and ventilatory support, blood pressure support, and control of arrhythmias.[8] In cases of severe bupivacaine toxicity, advanced life support is essential, and IV administration of lipid emulsion may provide an effective antidote.[9]

Recommended doses of commonly administered LAs are presented in **Table 9.1**.

α_2-Agonists

Alpha-2 (α_2) receptor agonists (eg, clonidine and dexmedetomidine) provide sedation, anxiolysis, and analgesia through central actions in the dorsal horn of the spinal cord and brainstem.[10-12] This combination of anxiolysis and potentiation of analgesia may be desirable for many patients recovering from major surgery. Coadministration of clonidine plus an opioid agonist produces more effective analgesia with a reduction in adverse effects than higher doses of either drug administered by itself. Premedication with oral or transdermal clonidine decreased morphine requirements when administered as part of a multimodal analgesic regimen.[13,14] IV clonidine reduced pain, nausea, and vomiting, and improved patient satisfaction with their pain relief.[10,11] This ability to potentiate opioid-mediated analgesia is particularly useful in patients with opioid tolerance or those highly sensitive to opioids.

Clonidine is available in oral, epidural, and transdermal formulations. Parenteral preparations are available for pain management in the European Union. Clonidine has excellent oral bioavailability, and dosing is equivalent to parenteral administration. Oral tablets

TABLE 9.1 — Onset and Duration of Local Anesthetic Action

	Onset (min)	Duration (hr)	Prolongation With Epinephrine	Toxic Dose With Single Administration
Ester				
Procaine	3-5	½-1	++	10-12 mg/kg
Chloroprocaine	10	½-1	++	10-12 mg/kg
Tetracaine	<15	2-3+	++	2 mg total
Benzocaine (topical)	<2	½+	++	200 mg total
Amide				
Lidocaine	<2	½-1	++	4-5 mg/kg (7 with epinephrine)
Bupivacaine	5	2-4	+/-	1.7-2 mg/kg
Mepivacaine	<5	¾-1½	++	4-5 mg/kg (7 with epinephrine)
Prilocaine	<2	1	?	8-10 mg/kg
Ropivacaine		1½-3	+/-	3 mg/kg
Bupivacaine liposomal injectable suspension	5	Up to 72	N/A	Safety data up to 532 mg

Key: ++, significant potentiation; +/-, some potentiation; N/A, not applicable.

are supplied in 0.1-mg, 0.2-mg, and 0.3-mg strengths. Starting doses of 2 mcg/kg/qd with titration up to 5 mcg/kg/qd are recommended. Transdermal patches release 0.2 mg clonidine per hour and are convenient for patients who cannot tolerate an oral diet. The patch is usually applied preoperatively or intraoperatively, since the onset of analgesic effect may be delayed 3 to 4 hours.

Perioperative administration of clonidine may be associated with alterations in hemodynamics, including an initial hypertensive phase followed by hypotension and bradycardia. Orthostatic hypotension can limit its safety in elderly and volume-depleted patients. Significant sedation can also occur with higher doses of clonidine. The initial hypertension phase is generally transient and should be treated cautiously with short-acting medications. Volume resuscitation and administration of ephedrine and atropine can be used to treat hypotension and bradycardia.

Dexmedetomidine is a more selective α_2-agonist than clonidine and has a shorter duration of action. Although not specifically approved for the treatment of postoperative pain, IV administration of dexmedetomidine was also associated with a 66% reduction in morphine use in the early postoperative period after major inpatient surgery.[15] Its use was associated with increased postoperative sedation and bradycardia.[16] As a result, patients receiving dexmedetomidine require monitoring in a PACU or telemetry setting.

Muscle Relaxants

The hyperalgesic response to acute surgical injury includes skeletal muscle spasm in dermatomes adjacent to site of incision and dissection.[14] Large muscle groups, including the rectus abdominus following abdominal surgery, the latissimus following flank incisions, and trapezius following cervical vertebral surgery, commonly undergo intense spasm that can be palpated by the surgeon and is a major source of patient discomfort. Accumulation of lactic acid in these muscle groups is very irritating to peripheral nociceptors and can elicit pain as intense as the incision itself. Hyperalgesic muscle spasm can also lead to splinting behavior that impedes pulmonary function, ambulation, and rehabilitation.[14] In general, opioids are ineffective in reversing muscle spasm or pain related to the spasm. Muscle relaxants are not primary analgesics but can be used to reduce skeletal muscle spasm and indirectly reduce splinting behavior and pain.[17,18]

Muscle relaxants have virtually no shared structure and no shared mechanism of action. Central-acting muscle relaxants are primarily CNS depressants, while others have activity at skeletal muscles or muscle spindles and are termed "direct muscle relaxants."[17,18] Methocarbamol (Robaxin) and carisoprodol (Soma) are examples of central sedatives that have secondary muscle relaxation effects. While effective, they have no direct action on the contractile mechanism of striated muscle or the motor end plate. These and other central-acting muscle relaxants are associated with dependency and abuse and should not be prescribed for prolonged periods of time. Carisoprodol has been ranked number 14 of the 20 most abused mood-altering drugs in the United States.[18]

Tricyclic analogues, including cyclobenzaprine (Flexeril), block 5-HT_2 receptors in the ventral spinal cord, thereby inhibiting the tonic α-motorneuron excitation produced by descending serotonergic nerve fibers.[19] A more recently developed muscle relaxant, tizanidine (Zanaflex), is an α_2-agonist that attenuates monosynaptic and polysynaptic motor reflexes in the spinal cord. Tizanidine decreases excitatory neurotransmitter release from small sensory afferents, and decreases activity of both α and γ motor neurons, reducing peripheral spasm. Tizanidine and cyclobenzaprine are commonly prescribed to patients discharged to home following laminectomy and spinal fusion.

Benzodiazepines such as diazepam (Valium) and lorazepam (Ativan) are muscle relaxants that are most commonly used for surgical inpatients.[20-22] These agents enhance the actions of GABA on its receptor and open inhibitory chloride ion channels.[21,22] The ability of benzodiazepines to block various neurophysiologic responses follows a specific dose-dependent order: antipanic> anticonvulsion> sedation> muscle relaxation.[21] This order explains why effective muscle relaxation is generally associated with antianxiety effects, as well as excessive sedation.

Oral and parenteral doses of diazepam have been approved for relief of muscle spasm. Oral doses range from 2 mg to 10 mg, three to four times daily (up to 30 mg/day). Parenteral doses range from 2 mg to 10 mg IV/IM every 4 to 6 hours. The half-life of diazepam ranges from approximately 24 hours to >48 hours.[22,23] The half-life is prolonged in the elderly and in patients with cirrhosis or hepatitis.[22]

While not approved for relief of muscle spasm, lorazepam is commonly prescribed for this condition, as well as for anxiety and insomnia. Oral doses range from 2 mg/day to 6 mg/day, given in two or three divided doses. Parenteral doses range from 2 mg/day to 6 mg/day, given in divided doses. Lorazepam is readily and completely absorbed from the GI tract after oral absorption. Peak plasma levels are reached at approximately 2 hours. Lorazepam has a longer therapeutic half-life than diazepam despite the fact that its elimination half-life is shorter (10 to 20 hours).

Side effects associated with diazepam and lorazepam include sedation, dizziness, weakness, unsteadiness, habituation, and memory impairment.[21-23] Diazepam, lorazepam, cyclobenzaprine, and tizanidine can be combined in multimodal fashion with oral steroids, opioids, and NSAIDs, based on the severity of symptoms. All muscle relaxants should be used cautiously in patients treated with opioids as they can enhance opioid-related respiratory depression and somnolence. Consider reducing opioid dose by 20% to 25% in patients coadministered muscle relaxants and benefiting from reductions in muscle spasm–related pain.

Anticonvulsant Analgesics

Anticonvulsant analgesics, such as gabapentin (Neurontin) and pregabalin (Lyrica), can effectively control neuropathic pain and are approved for use in patients with:

- Postherpetic neuralgia
- Fibromyalgia
- Diabetic neuropathy.

While not indicated for surgical pain management, they are increasingly prescribed in this setting.[14]

Gabapentin was initially approved for control of partial seizures in adults.[24] Soon after its release, a number of uncontrolled trials were published attesting to its safety and effectiveness in patients with postherpetic neuralgia, trigeminal neuralgia, and reflex sympathetic dystrophy.[25] A more recently approved gabapentinoid, pregabalin, was conceived and developed as an antineuropathic analgesic.[26] Pregabalin has neurochemical and therapeutic similarities to gabapentin but is more selective, has greater tolerability, and is simpler to dose.

9

Gabapentin and pregabalin exhibit high binding affinity at the α_2–δ subunit of presynaptic voltage-gated calcium channels.[27] Their analgesic effects may be related to inhibition of calcium influx and diminished release of excitatory neurotransmitters in spinal and supraspinal pain pathways. Gabapentin and pregabalin also reduce the excitability of irritated and injured peripheral noxious fibers. Common side effects observed with a therapeutic dose are dizziness and sedation, which are often tolerable if the dose is started low.

In addition to their use in chronic pain, both gabapentin and pregabalin offer therapeutic options for acute pain and have been advocated for use as perioperative analgesic adjuvants.[28-30] Pre- and postoperative doses of gabapentin (900 mg) and pregabalin (150 mg) have been shown to reduce opioid consumption in several postsurgical models. Gabapentin and pregabalin appear to be more effective in surgical procedures associated with acute nerve injury rather than inflammatory pain. They do not improve acute pain intensity scores, but both have been shown to reduce wound-site hyperalgesia.

Zhang and coworkers recently performed a meta-analysis of pregabalin as an adjuvant for postsurgical pain.[31] Doses of 300 mg/day did not reduce pain intensity during the first 24 hours following surgery but did significantly decrease opioid consumption during this interval (**Figure 9.3**). Patients treated with pregabalin benefited from less nausea and vomiting but reported a higher incidence of visual disturbances. Perioperative administration of anticonvulsant analgesics may also reduce central sensitization and the development of persistent pain. Fassoulaki and colleagues[32] evaluated the benefits of gabapentin (400 mg tid) in women undergoing mastectomy. Patients treated with gabapentin required less postoperative acetaminophen and opioids than did the controls. Of greater importance was the finding that at 3 and 6 months following surgery, 10 of 22 patients treated with gabapentin (45%) reported chronic pain as compared with 18 of 22 untreated controls (82%) (P<0.02). None of the 22 patients treated with gabapentin required opioids at 6 months vs five of 22 controls (P<0.107).

When employed as analgesic adjuvants for postsurgical pain, the following doses are recommended:

- Gabapentin 600 mg to 900 mg preoperatively, followed by 600 mg to 900 mg tid for 24 to 72 hours
- Pregabalin 75 mg to 150 mg preoperatively, followed by 75mg to 150 mg bid for 24 to 72 hours.

Both drugs are cleared by the kidneys; hence, dosage should be reduced significantly in patients with renal impairment.

FIGURE 9.3 — 24-Hour Morphine Consumption (mg) in Postsurgical Patients Receiving Pregabalin <300 mg/day

Study or Subgroup	Pregabalin Mean	Pregabalin SD	Pregabalin Total	Control Mean	Control SD	Control Total	Weight (%)	Mean Difference IV, Randomization, 95% CI	Mean Difference IV, Randomization, 95% CI
Agarwal and colleagues, 150 mg	55.52	12.48	27	75.75	9.93	29	24.1	-20.23 (-26.16, -14.30)	
Jokela and colleagues, 150 mg	17.3	10.2	26	18.6	10.7	28	24.5	-1.30 (-6.87, 4.27)	
Jokela and colleagues, 75 mg	16.3	7.7	30	18.6	10.7	28	25.3	-2.30 (-7.13, 2.53)	
Cabrera Schulmeyer and colleagues, 150 mg	11.51	7.93	39	23.07	9.57	41	26.2	-11.56 (-15.40, -7.72)	
Total (95% CI)			**122**			**126**	**100.0%**	**-8.80 (-16.65, -0.94)**	

Heterogeneity: $\tau^2 = 57.51$; $\chi^2 = 30.15$, df = 3 (P <0.00001); $I^2 = 90\%$

Test for overall effect: $Z = 2.20$ ($P = 0.03$)

Modified from Zhang J, et al. *Br J Anaesth*. 2011;106(4):454-462.

NMDA Receptor Antagonists (Ketamine)

Ketamine (2-(O-chlorophenyl)-2-methylamino cyclohexanone) is a nonopioid, central-acting dissociative anesthetic. At subanesthetic doses, ketamine provides rapid and highly potent analgesia without many of the serious adverse effects observed with opioids.[14] Although ketamine's exact mechanism of action remains unclear, several hypotheses have been proposed to explain its clinical effect. Ketamine binds and antagonizes NMDA receptors in the CNS. It also provides analgesia by interacting with σ-opiate receptors at the spinal and central level, and by activation of phencyclidine receptors.[33,34]

Ketamine potentiates opioid-mediated analgesia and provides a significant opioid-sparing effect.[13,33,34] Measurable reductions in the opioid dose requirement can reduce the incidence of annoying side effects such as nausea, vomiting, and oversedation, as well as life-threatening adverse effects such as respiratory depression. A commonly used approach is to provide a ketamine infusion as an adjunct for IV-PCA with morphine or hydromorphone. A continuous ketamine infusion of 0.1 to 0.2 mg/kg/hour and up to 2 mg/kg/day provides useful augmentation of opioid PCA with minimal to no adverse effects (**Table 9.2**). Ketamine can also be administered directly via a PCA device. PCA solutions may be formulated with ketamine and morphine in a 1:1 ratio. Patient boluses of 0.5 mg morphine plus 0.5 mg ketamine every 6 to 8 minutes are as effective as boluses with higher-concentration morphine (1 mg) every 6 to 8 minutes.

Ketamine has particular utility in opioid-tolerant patients. Urban and colleagues[35] performed a prospective randomized study to assess the use of ketamine (0.2 mg/kg on induction of general anesthesia, then 2 mcg/kg/hour for the next 24 hours) vs placebo as an adjunct to IV-PCA hydromorphone in 26 opioid-tolerant patients undergoing spinal fusions.

TABLE 9.2 — Ketamine for Supplementation of Postsurgical Analgesia

Intraoperative	Postoperative
Bolus 0.2-0.3 mg/kg at anesthetic induction	Initiate infusion 0.1 mg/kg/hr in PACU; maintain for 24-72 hours as required[a]
OR	
Bolus 0.1 mg/kg at anesthetic induction, then initiate infusion 0.1 mg/kg/hr and maintain for 24-72 hours as required	Maintain infusion 0.1 mg/kg/hr for 24-72 hours as required[a]

[a] Infusion may be increased to 0.2 mg/kg/hr or more in selected patients. Side effects, including agitation, auditory and visual hallucinations, and tremor, increase in incidence and severity with increasing ketamine dose. Judicious administration of valium and ativan may reduce the severity of side effects. Avoid ketamine in patients with histories of severe rate-related coronary or valvular heart disease, raised intracranial pressure, and seizures.

Coadministration of ketamine resulted in significantly less pain in the PACU during the first postoperative day and during physical therapy. Patients in the ketamine group required significantly less hydromorphone than the control group.

Elia and Tramer[36] performed a meta-analysis that evaluated ketamine for postoperative pain. They reported that low-dose IV ketamine decreased postoperative pain intensity up to 48 hours, decreased cumulative 24-hour morphine consumption, and delayed the time to first request for rescue analgesic. Similar results were obtained regarding the use of ketamine in a 2006 Cochrane analysis.[33]

Major complications associated with ketamine include hyperdynamic cardiovascular responses and psychomimetic reactions. Relative contraindications to bolus dosing include patients with uncontrolled hypertension, congestive heart failure, tachyarrhythmias, myocardial ischemia, head and globe injuries, and increased intracranial pressure.[35] It is unclear whether low-dose infusions are absolutely contraindicated in all of these settings. Low-dose infusions (0.1 mg/kg/hour) are associated with an improved CNS tolerability profile, although a small number of patients may experience diplopia, mild hallucinations, and confusion.

Corticosteroids

Oral corticosteroids offer potent anti-inflammatory effects that may reduce the intensity of postsurgical pain. Glucocorticoids bind to specific cytoplasmic and nuclear receptors in injured cells, thereby stabilizing lysosomal membranes and preventing the release of destructive acid hydrolases.[37] The anti-inflammatory actions of glucocorticoids involve suppression of phospholipase A_2 and arachidonic acid release, as well as reductions in the synthesis of prostaglandins and leukotrienes. Reductions in inflammation and edema are especially beneficial in controlling bone pain, compressive neuropathic pain, and pain from bowel obstruction and organ capsule distention.[37] In addition to these anti-inflammatory effects, oral corticosteroids promote gluconeogenesis, reduce nausea and vomiting, stimulate the appetite, and lead to a sense of well-being.

The analgesic effect of glucocorticoids has been well documented, especially in the postoperative setting. Peak analgesic potency appears comparable to that provided by optimal doses of NSAIDs and acetaminophen, although the onset of clinical effect is delayed. In patients treated with 16 mg IV dexamethasone following recovery from breast surgery, analgesic effects were not observed until 4 hours postdose.[38] On the other hand, the duration of analgesia provided by single IV doses of glucocorticoid may be prolonged for up to 3 days. In ambulatory surgical settings, patients treated with a single dose of IV ketorolac experienced a rapid onset of analgesia, while those treated with methylprednisolone generally report more pain in the PACU, but require less rescue analgesics during postoperative days 2 and 3.[37] Prednisone and dexamethasone are rapidly absorbed across the GI mucosa following oral administration but may be given parenterally to patients not tolerating oral diets. The optimal glucocorticoid analgesic dose is not established, as controlled dose-finding studies have not been performed. Dexamethasone doses of 3 mg to 4 mg provide useful antiemetic effects, although doses as high as 8 mg to 12 mg may be required to gain effective analgesia.[38] The combination of a glucocorticoid plus an NSAID provides additive anti-inflammatory effects and analgesia.[39]

For patients with known contraindications to NSAIDs, glucocorticoids may offer a safe and useful substitute. In a meta-analysis focused on risk and benefits, no significant side effects were found in 17 studies (941 patients) utilizing single doses of dexamethasone.[40] A second meta-analysis of higher-dose methylprednisolone (ie, 15 mg/kg to 30 mg/kg) in over 2000 chest trauma patients also found no significant adverse effects.[41] Nonbeneficial effects may occur with prolonged glucocorticoid use, including osteoporosis and spontaneous fractures, avascular necrosis of bone, muscle wasting, psychotic reactions, hyperglycemia, and peptic ulceration. Corticosteroids should not be administered to patients with active herpes simplex keratitis, vaccinia, varicella, mycobacterial, and systemic fungal infections, active peptic ulcer disease, or nonspecific ulcerative colitis.

Tricyclic Antidepressants

TCAs have also been advocated as analgesic adjuvants for postsurgical pain.[14] While this class of drugs was originally developed to manage depression, TCAs were found to effectively control neuropathic pain, fibromyalgia, and neck and low back pain.[42] Mechanisms underlying the analgesic activity of TCAs remain unclear but appear to be distinct from their antidepressant properties. TCAs inhibit presynaptic reuptake proteins, decrease serotonin and norepinephrine reuptake, and increase norepinephrine concentrations in spinal cord and brainstem. Norepinephrine binds to and activates postsynaptic α-adrenergic receptors, thereby suppressing pain transmission.[42,43] Analgesic effects are achieved more rapidly and with lower doses than for antidepressant effects. Traditionally, the tertiary amine amitriptyline (Elavil) has been favored for acute pain management over nortriptyline.[44,45]

It should be appreciated that TCAs are not approved for any pain indications, although amitriptyline has been advocated for postsurgical pain control as well as nighttime sedation. TCAs are most effective for surgical procedures associated with neural trauma and postoperative neuropathic symptoms. These include amputation and traumatic or surgical injuries to the intercostal nerves, branches of the brachial plexus, and inguinal and genitofemoral nerves. The surgeon should consider starting doses of 12.5 mg to 25 mg and increase to 50 mg as tolerated.[42,43]

TCAs offer several advantages for selected patient populations when used for multimodal analgesia. They are not narcotics and are nonhabituating, are inexpensive, easily prescribed, and widely available in pharmacies and hospital formularies. Use caution when using TCAs in patients treated with MAOIs, SSRIs, cimetidine, haloperidol, or phenothiazines. Also use caution when drugs that lower the seizure threshold, prolong the QT interval, or have anticholinergic properties are coadministered.[42] Monitor for blurred vision, orthostatic hypotension, urinary retention, and constipation. Less caution may be needed with low-dose administration (12.5 mg to 25 mg). Sedation and dry mouth are commonly observed. For this reason, it is best to administer TCAs at bedtime where they may help to improve sleep. Common adverse events observed with TCAs are presented in **Table 9.3**.

REFERENCES

1. Practice guidelines for acute pain management in the perioperative setting. A report by the American Society of Anesthesiologists Task Force on Pain Management, Acute Pain Section. *Anesthesiology*. 1995;82(4):1071-1081.

2. Butterworth J. Local anesthetics in regional anesthesia and acute pain management. In: Sinatra R, de Leon-Casasola O, Ginsberg B, Viscusi E, eds. *Acute Pain Management.* New York, NY: Cambridge University Press; 2009:70-81.

3. Strichartz GR, Sanchez V, Arthur GR, Chafetz R, Martin D. Fundamental properties of local anesthetics. II. Measured octanol:buffer partition coefficients and pKa values of clinically used drugs. *Anesth Analg*. 1990;71(2):158-170.

4. Butterworth J, Ririe DG, Thompson RB, Walker FO, Jackson D, James RL. Differential onset of median nerve block: randomized, double-blind comparison of mepivacaine and bupivacaine in healthy volunteers. *Br J Anaesth*. 1998;81(4):515-521.

5. Whiteman A, Bajaj S, Hasan M. Novel techniques of local anaesthetic infiltration. *Contin Educ Anaesth Crit Care Pain*. 2011;11(5):167-171.

6. Ilfeld BM, Morey TE, Thannikary LJ, Wright TW, Enneking FK. Clonidine added to a continuous interscalene ropivacaine perineural infusion to improve postoperative analgesia: a randomized, double-blind, controlled study. *Anesth Analg*. 2005;100(4):1172-1178.

7. Mather LE, Copeland SE, Ladd LA. Acute toxicity of local anesthetics: underlying pharmacokinetic and pharmacodynamic concepts. *Reg Anesth Pain Med*. 2005;30(6):553-566.

8. Rosenblatt MA, Abel M, Fischer GW, Itzkovich CJ, Eisenkraft JB. Successful use of a 20% lipid emulsion to resuscitate a patient after a presumed bupivacaine-related cardiac arrest. *Anesthesiology*. 2006;105(1):217-218.

9. Bigat Z, Boztug N, Hadiminglu N, Cete N, Coskunfirat N, Ertok E. Does dexamethasone improve the quality of intravenous regional anesthesia and analgesia? A randomized, controlled clinical study. *Anesth Analg*. 2006;102(2):605-609.

10. Micromedex Healthcare Series. *DrugDex Evaluations. Clonidine.* New York, NY: Thompson Healthcare.

11. Hayashi Y, Guo TZ, Maze M. Desensitization to the behavioral effects of alpha 2-adrenergic agonists in rats. *Anesthesiology*. 1995;82(4):954-962.

TABLE 9.3 — Tricyclic Antidepressants: Side Effect Profile

			Side Effects					
			α-1 Blockade	**Cholinergic Blockade**	**Dopamine Blockade**	**Histamine Blockade**	**NE Reuptake Blockade**	**5-HT Reuptake Blockade**
Generic (Trade) Name	**Formulations (mg)**	**Maximum Daily Dose (mg)**	• Orthostatic hypotension • Dizziness • Tachycardia	• Blurred vision • Dry mouth • Memory loss • Urinary retention • Constipation	• EPS • Prolactin elevation	• Sedation • Weight gain	• Sweating • Anxiety	• Diarrhea • Nausea
Tertiary Amine								
Amitriptyline (Elavil) (active metabolite: nortriptyline)	Tablet: 10, 25, 50, 75, 100, 150 Parenteral: 10 mg/mL	300	++++	++++	+	+++	++	++

Secondary Amine								
Nortriptyline (Pamelor)	Capsule: 10, 25, 50, 75 Oral solution: 10 mg/5 mL	150	+++	++	+	++	+++	+/-

Key: +/-, minimal; ++, some; +++, significant, ++++, highly significant.

9

12. Jeffs SA, Hall JE, Morris S. Comparison of morphine alone with morphine plus clonidine for postoperative patient-controlled analgesia. *Br J Anaesth*. 2002;89(3):424-427.

13. Singh H, Liu J, Gaines GY, White PF. Effect of oral clonidine and intrathecal fentanyl on tetracaine spinal block. *Anesth Analg*. 1994;79(6):1113-1116.

14. Knotkova H, Pappagallo M. Adjuvant analgesics. *Anesthesiol Clin*. 2007;25(4):775-786.

15. Arain SR, Ruehlow RM, Uhrich TD, Ebert TJ. The efficacy of dexmedetomidine versus morphine for postoperative analgesia after major inpatient surgery. *Anesth Analg*. 2004;98(1):153-158.

16. Precedex (dexmedetomidine hydrochloride) injection [package insert]. Lake Forest, IL: Hospira, Inc; 2010.

17. Chou R, Peterson K, Helfand M. Comparative efficacy and safety of skeletal muscle relaxants for spasticity and musculoskeletal conditions: a systematic review. *J Pain Symptom Manage*. 2004;28(2):140-175.

18. Toth PP, Urtis J. Commonly used muscle relaxant therapies for acute low back pain: a review of carisoprodol, cyclobenzaprine hydrochloride, and metaxalone. *Clin Ther*. 2004;26(9):1355-1367.

19. Honda M, Nishida T, Ono H. Tricyclic analogs cyclobenzaprine, amitriptyline and cyproheptadine inhibit the spinal reflex transmission through 5-HT(2) receptors. *Eur J Pharmacol*. 2003;458(1-2):91-99.

20. Schmidt RT, Lee RH, Spehlmann R. Comparison of dantrolene sodium and diazepam in the treatment of spasticity. *J Neurol Neurosurg Psychiatry*. 1976;39(4):350-356.

21. Valium (diazepam) [package insert]. Nutley, NJ: Roche Laboratories Inc; January 2008.

22. Haefely W, Kyburz E, Gerecke M, et al. Recent advances in the molecular pharmacology of benzodiazepine receptors and in the structure-activity relationships of their agonists and antagonists. In: Testa B, ed. *Advances in Drug Research.* Vol 14. London, England: Academic Press; 1985:165-322.

23. Sieghart W. Pharmacology of benzodiazepine receptors: an update. *J Psychiatry Neurosci*. 1994;19(1):24-29.

24. Goa KL, Sorkin EM. Gabapentin. A review of its pharmacological properties and clinical potential in epilepsy. *Drugs*. 1993;46(3):409-427.

25. Mellick GA, Mellicy LB, Mellick LB. Gabapentin in the management of reflex sympathetic dystrophy. *J Pain Symptom Manage*. 1995;10(4):265-266.

26. Lyrica (pregabalin) [package insert]. New York, NY: Pfizer; June 2011.

27. Luo ZD, Calcutt NA, Higuera ES, et al. Injury type-specific calcium channel alpha 2 delta-1 subunit up-regulation in rat neuropathic pain models correlates with antiallodynic effects of gabapentin. *J Pharmacol Exp Ther*. 2002;303(3):1199-1205.

28. Gilron I, Orr E, Tu D, O'Neill JP, Zamora JE, Bell AC. A placebo-controlled randomized clinical trial of perioperative administration of gabapentin, rofecoxib and their combination for spontaneous and movement-evoked pain after abdominal hysterectomy. *Pain*. 2005;113(1-2):191-200.

29. Dahl JB, Mathiesen O, Møiniche S. 'Protective premedication': an option with gabapentin and related drugs? A review of gabapentin and pregabalin in the treatment of post-operative pain. *Acta Anaesthesiol Scand*. 2004;48(9):1130-1136.

30. Durkin B, Page C, Glass P. Pregabalin for the treatment of post-surgical pain. *Expert Opin Pharmacother*. 2010;11(16):2751-2758.

31. Zhang J, Ho KY, Wang Y. Efficacy of pregabalin in acute post-operative pain: a meta-analysis. *Br J Anaesth*. 2011;106(4):454-462.

32. Fassoulaki A, Triga A, Melemeni A, Sarantopoulos C. Multimodal analgesia with gabapentin and local anesthetics prevents acute and chronic pain after breast surgery for cancer. *Anesth Analg*. 2005;101(5):1427-1432.

33. Bell RF, Dahl JB, Moore RA, Kalso E. Perioperative ketamine for acute postoperative pain. *Cochrane Database Syst Rev*. 2006;(1):CD004603.

34. De Kock M, Lavand'homme P, Waterloos H. 'Balanced analgesia' in the perioperative period: is there a place for ketamine? *Pain*. 2001;92(3):373-380.

35. Urban MK, Ya Deau JT, Wukovits B, Lipnitsky JY. Ketamine as an adjunct to postoperative pain management in opioid tolerant patients after spinal fusions: a prospective randomized trial. *HSS J*. 2008;4(1):62-65.

36. Elia N, Tramèr MR. Ketamine and postoperative pain--a quantitative systematic review of randomised trials. *Pain*. 2005;113(1-2):61-70.

37. Raeder J, Dahl V. Clinical application of glucocorticoids, antineuropathics, and other analgesic adjuvants for acute pain management. In: Sinatra R, de Leon-Casasola O, Ginsberg B, Viscusi E, eds. *Acute Pain Management*. New York, NY; Cambridge University Press; 2009:377-390.

38. Romundstad L, Breivik H, Niemi G, Helle A, Stubhaug A. Methylprednisolone intravenously 1 day after surgery has sustained analgesic and opioid-sparing effects. *Acta Anaesthesiol Scand*. 2004;48(10):1223-1231.

39. Karst M, Kegel T, Lukas A, Lüdemann W, Hussein S, Piepenbrock S. Effect of celecoxib and dexamethasone on postoperative pain after lumbar disc surgery. *Neurosurgery*. 2003;53(2):331-336.

40. Salerno A, Hermann R. Efficacy and safety of steroid use for postoperative pain relief. Update and review of the medical literature. *J Bone Joint Surg Am*. 2006;88(6):1361-1372.

41. Abdi S, Datta S, Trescot AM, et al. Epidural steroids in the management of chronic spinal pain: a systematic review. *Pain Physician*. 2007;10(1):185-212.

42. McQuay HJ, Moore RA. Antidepressants and chronic pain. *BMJ*. 1997;314(7083):763-764.

43. O'Connor AB, Noyes K, Holloway RG. A cost-effectiveness comparison of desipramine, gabapentin, and pregabalin for treating postherpetic neuralgia. *J Am Geriatr Soc*. 2007;55 (8):1176-1184.

44. Kerrick JM, Fine PG, Lipman AG, Love G. Low-dose amitriptyline as an adjunct to opioids for postoperative orthopedic pain: a placebo-controlled trial. *Pain*. 1993;52(3):325-330.

45. Robinson LR, Czerniecki JM, Ehde DM, et al. Trial of amitriptyline for relief of pain in amputees: results of a randomized controlled study. *Arch Phys Med Rehabil*. 2004;85(1):1-6.

10 Acetaminophen

by Raymond S. Sinatra, MD, PhD

Introduction

Acetaminophen (also known as paracetamol and APAP) is a synthetic central-acting analgesic for mild-to-moderate acute and chronic pain.[1-3] Unlike NSAIDs, acetaminophen is not a peripheral-acting analgesic and has negligible COX inhibitory and anti-inflammatory effects at the site of surgical injury.[2,3] Acetaminophen is recommended as a first-line analgesic in mild-to-moderate acute pain states and is effective in combination with opioids and other analgesics for more severe pain. Acetaminophen's exact mechanism of analgesic effect is not clearly understood. It is believed to activate descending serotonergic inhibitory pathways. This interaction is indirect and not associated with binding to serotonin receptors.[2-4] Acetaminophen is an inhibitor of central COX-2 and possibly COX-3, and has been shown to decrease prostaglandin synthesis in the spinal cord and brainstem. One of the metabolites (AM404) has cannabinoid agonist activity and inhibits TRPV-1 ion channels in pain-conducting pathways.[5] Acetaminophen directly inhibits the hypothalamic heat-regulating center, resulting in peripheral vasodilatation and increased dissipation of heat.[1-3]

Oral and Rectal Formulations

Acetaminophen was discovered in 1879, yet widespread distribution and use of oral acetaminophen (Tylenol) in the United States and paracetamol (Panadol) in Europe did not occur until the 1950s. It has since become the most widely administered over-the-counter analgesic worldwide.[1-3] In addition, opioid compounds containing acetaminophen (eg, Percocet, Tylox, Vicodin, Lortab) are also the most widely prescribed analgesics for the management of post-surgical pain. Both oral and rectal acetaminophen are commonly utilized to treat mild-to-moderately severe incisional and musculoskeletal pain after ambulatory surgery.

Standard oral and rectal doses for short-term use (1 to 5 days) are 325 mg to 650 mg every 4 hours or 1000 mg three to four times per day, with a maximum of 4000 mg/day. Thereafter, the maximum dose should be reduced to 3200 mg/day.[2-3] In pediatric patients, the recommended rectal dose is 15 mg/kg every 6 hours (40-60 mg/kg/day). This dose has been shown to significantly reduce morphine requirements in children recovering from day surgery procedures.[6] A meta-analysis that assessed 51 double-blind, placebo-controlled trials of oral acetaminophen found that significantly more patients experienced a 50% reduction in postsurgical pain over 4 to 6 hours compared with placebo (50% vs 20%).[7]

In recommended doses, acetaminophen does not irritate the lining of the stomach, inhibit platelet aggregation, or affect kidney function as do NSAIDs. Unlike aspirin, acetaminophen is safe in children as it is not associated with a risk of Reye's syndrome in those with viral illnesses. In contrast to opioids, acetaminophen is not associated with nausea, vomiting, and constipation, nor does it alter mood or pose a risk of dependency, tolerance, or withdrawal.[1,2]

Intravenous Acetaminophen

Intravenous formulations of acetaminophen (IV-acetaminophen) were developed in Europe in the 1980s specifically for postsurgical pain management and control of fever in patients unable to tolerate oral dosing. An early preparation, IV propacetamol, was associated with burning at the injection site and was replaced by IV paracetamol (Perfalgan), which provided greater stability and fewer adverse events.[8,9] Significant advantages were offered by IV-acetaminophen over oral/rectal routes, including:

- A more rapid and more predictable onset
- Higher maximum plasma concentration
- Higher analgesic efficacy.

It has become the most widely administered nonopioid analgesic in the European Union, with over 400 million doses administered since 2002.[9,10] Subseqently, IV-acetaminophen was evaluated in several clinical trials in the United States and gained FDA approval for clinical use in 2010.

Currently, IV-acetaminophen (Ofirmev) is approved for:

- Management of mild-to-moderate pain
- Management of moderate-to-severe pain with adjunctive opioid analgesics
- Reduction of fever in adult and pediatric patients.[11]

It is available in a 1-g/100-mL glass infusion bottle, contents of which do not require reconstitution. The solution should not be bolused rapidly but rather infused via peripheral IV over a period of 15 minutes. The recommended dose for adults weighing ≥50 kg is 1000 mg every 4 to 6 hours, with a maximum of 4000 mg/day, and no adjustment in dosage is necessary for patients up to 70 years of age weighing >50 kg. As a result of changes in volume of distribution in patients >80 years of age, the area under the curve (AUC) of acetaminophen plasma concentration is 54% to 68% higher than in adults <60 years of age.[12] The elimination half-life is slightly prolonged (2.7 to 3.2 hours in 70- to 80-year-old patients, and 3.6 hours in 80- to 90-year-old patients). These findings suggest a dose adjustment for IV-acetaminophen of 650 mg to 750 mg every 6 hours in these age groups. The recommended dose for children and adolescents weighing <50 kg, is 15 mg/kg every 4 to 6 hours, with a maximum of 3 g/day.[11]

In the perioperative setting, IV-acetaminophen offers several advantages, particularly in patients who are unable to tolerate oral medications or in those with unpredictable GI function.[9,10] IV administration achieves maximal plasma concentrations (T_{max}) more rapidly and predictably than that observed with oral and rectal dosing. Maximum plasma concentration of drug (C_{max}) following a 15-minute IV-acetaminophen infusion was significantly higher than that observed with similar doses given orally[13] (**Figure 10.1**). No accumulation of drug is noted with repeated doses given every 6 hours. In clinical trials, IV-acetaminophen is superior to oral acetaminophen and comparable to IV ketorolac 30 mg for the treatment of moderate postsurgical pain.[9,10] Onset of analgesia with IV-acetaminophen occurs within 5 to 10 minutes, peak analgesic effect is noted at 1 hour, and its duration of effect is approximately 4 to 6 hours. The onset of its antipyretic effect occurs within 30 minutes, with a duration of 6 hours.[14]

In a trial of 151 patients with moderate-to-severe pain after orthopedic surgery, IV-acetaminophen (1 g) resulted in significantly better pain relief from 15 minutes to 6 hours postsurgically when compared with placebo[15] (**Figure 10.2**). In addition, the need for rescue IV-PCA morphine was delayed in patients receiving acetaminophen (3 hours vs 0.8 hours) and 24-hour morphine requirements were reduced by 33% (33.8 vs 57.4). The incidence of adverse events was significantly lower in the IV-acetaminophen group (8%) than in the placebo group (17%).

IV-acetaminophen was also evaluated for pain management following abdominal laparoscopic surgery. Patients were randomized to receive either IV-acetaminophen 1000 mg every 6 hours, IV-acetaminophen 650 mg every 4 hours, or placebo over 24 hours. The summed pain intensity differences (total reduction from baseline VAS scores) and subjective pain ratings over the first 24 hours were superior in the 1000-mg and 650-mg IV-acetaminophen groups when compared with placebo. There were no

FIGURE 10.1 — Pharmacokinetics of IV vs PO Acetaminophen

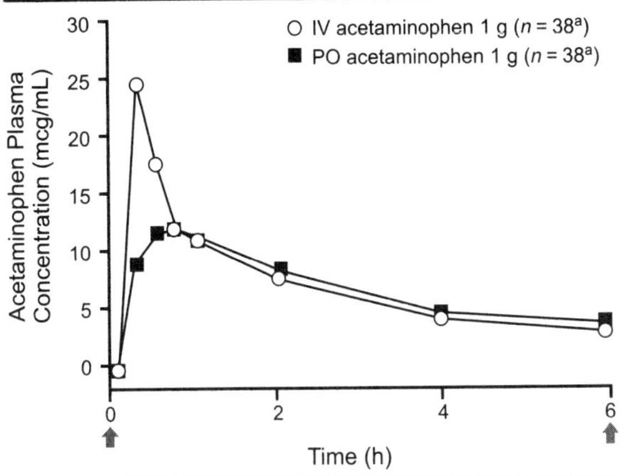

Mean acetaminophen concentration over time: 6-hour dosing regimen *(arrows)* of IV or PO acetaminophen in healthy adults.[1]

C_{max} is up to 70% higher in IV than in PO acetaminophen.[1,2] Overal exposures (AUC) are very similar for IV and PO acetaminophen.[2]

IV acetaminophen accumulation is similar to that of PO acetaminophen.[1]

[a] Of the 38 randomly assigned patients, 34 patients who received IV acetaminophen 1 g and 33 patients who received PO acetaminophen 1 g had plasma concentrations measured.

[b] Rapid-release liquid PO acetaminophen.

[1] Data on file Cadence Pharmaceuticals, Inc.

[2] Ofirmev [package insert]. San Diego, CA: Cadence Pharmaceuticals, Inc.; 2010.

differences in the incidence of serious adverse events or alterations in liver enzymes between treatment groups.[16]

The analgesic effectiveness of IV-acetaminophen for postsurgical pain management appears to be enhanced when administered prior to surgical incision. Using a preemptive analgesia protocol, Arici

FIGURE 10.2 — Pain Relief Scores in Patients Recovering From Major Orthopedic Surgery[1]

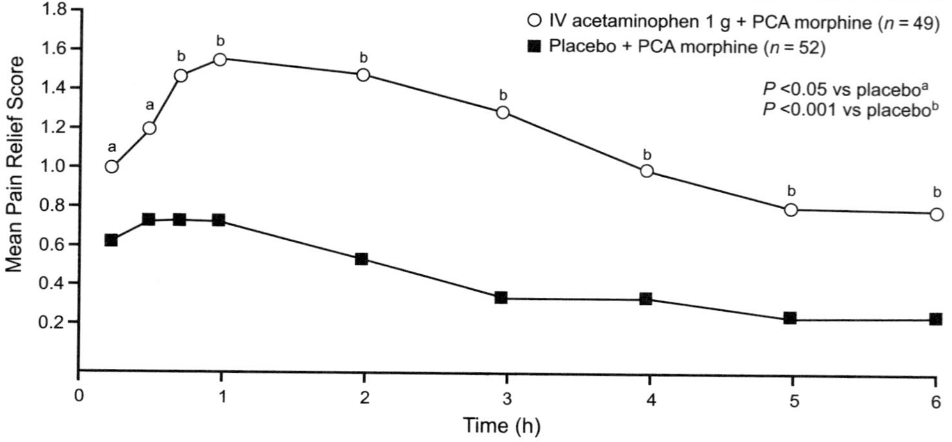

Mean Pain Relief Score

1.8
1.6
1.4
1.2
1.0
0.8
0.6
0.4
0.2

0 1 2 3 4 5 6

Time (h)

○ IV acetaminophen 1 g + PCA morphine ($n = 49$)
■ Placebo + PCA morphine ($n = 52$)

P <0.05 vs placebo[a]
P <0.001 vs placebo[b]

	IV Acetaminophen	Placebo	*P* value
Patient satisfaction: good to excellent at 24 hours	40.8%	23.1%	0.004[a,2]
Median time to first use of rescue	3.0 hours	0.8 hours	0.0001
Morphine consumption over 24 hours[b]	38.3 mg (33% ↓)	57.4 mg	<0.01
Safety (adverse reacations)	IV-acetaminophen is comparable with placebo		

[a] Based on Cochran-Mantel Haenszel test.
[b] Clinical benefit of reduced opioid consumption was not demonstrated.

[1] Sinatra RS, et al. *Anesthesiology*. 2005;102(4):822-831.
[2] Data on file Cadence Pharmaceuticals, Inc.

10

and colleagues[17] randomized 90 patients undergoing total abdominal hysterectomy to receive IV-acetaminophen (1 g) given 30 minutes prior to induction, IV-acetaminophen (1 g) given prior to skin closure, or IV saline. During the first 24 hours following surgery, morphine consumption was lowest in the preoperative IV-acetaminophen group (25.93 ± 5.69 mg) than the postsurgical IV-acetaminophen group (35.73 ± 5.24 mg). Morphine requirements were significantly higher in the placebo group (62.93 ± 8.67 mg) than either of the IV-acetaminophen groups. To date, over 22 double-blind randomized trials have demonstrated improvements in analgesic efficacy and opioid-dose sparing. Results of several key studies are summarized in **Table 10.1**.

Clinical Advantages

IV-acetaminophen offers several clinical advantages for perioperative use:

- It is well tolerated when employed as either analgesic monotherapy or as a multimodal adjunct.
- IV-acetaminophen is not associated with excessive sedation, biliary spasm, respiratory depression, nausea, vomiting, ileus, or pruritus observed with opioids.
- It is not associated with the harmful GI, hematologic, cardiovascular, or renal effects associated with NSAIDs and COX-2 inhibitors.[9,10]
- IV administration is associated with a more rapid onset and onset-to-peak analgesic effect and is more suitable for titrating and reducing the intensity of postsurgical pain.

Achieving earlier and higher plasma and CSF levels is most likely responsible for the rapid and surprisingly high analgesic efficacy of the IV preparation compared with what surgeons have come to expect with oral acetaminophen.[18] As there is no contraindication to preemptive dosing, effective blood concentrations of IV-acetaminophen can be achieved intraoperatively prior to emergence from anesthesia. We recommend that the infusion be initiated, as part of standard protocol, in the holding area immediately following placement of the peripheral IV catheter. The IV-acetaminophen bottle can be spiked and piggy-backed into the main IV line delivering standard lactated Ringer's or sodium chloride solution. Alternatively, the drug can be started by the anesthesiologist, ideally prior to initiation of neural blockade or induction of general anesthesia. If this is not possible, IV-acetaminophen can be started anytime during the procedure or upon patient arrival in the PACU.

Since IV-acetaminophen is a central-acting analgesic without anti-inflammatory effects, it may be combined with an NSAID or coxib to gain additive multimodal analgesic effects.[19] This additivity may be of particular benefit in patients recovering from colectomy or those presenting with histories of opioid-induced constipation. The combination of central and peripheral analgesic effects can further reduce opioid consumption and potential dose-dependent inhibition of bowel function.

■ Hepatic Toxicity

The main concern with any form of acetaminophen dosing is hepatic toxicity. Acetaminophen has a narrow therapeutic window, and even minor overdoses may cause severe hepatic injury. Liver necrosis occurs at 7.5 g to 10 g of acetaminophen. For this reason, it is important not to administer IV-acetaminophen in doses higher than the maximum recommended. IV-acetaminophen is contraindicated in patients with severe hepatic impairment or severe active liver disease. Pharmacokinetic modeling suggests that IV-acetaminophen may have a reduced risk of hepatotoxicity when compared with oral dosing, as it is not associated with high GI first-pass delivery to the liver. It is reassuring to know that hepatotoxicity does not occur when recommended doses of IV-acetaminophen are administered to healthy patients.

TABLE 10.1 — Randomized, Controlled Trials With IV Acetaminophen for Postsurgical Pain

Surgery	Patients	Treatment	Anesthesia	Treatment	Scale	Outcome
Orthopedic[1] adults 22-87	Hospitalized 1 g IV APAP vs years old	2 g PROP vs PBO	General	Given postop q6h × 24h	VAS, VRS	IV APAP significantly reduced pain and morphine consumption over 24-h period
Tonsillectomy[2]	Ambulatory adults 16-40 years old	1 g IV APAP vs PBO	General	Given postop q6h × 24h	VAS	IV APAP signficantly reduced meperidine consumption over 24-h period
Cardiac surgery[3]	Adults 45-79 years old	1 g IV APAP vs PBO	General	15 min before end of surgery and q6h × 72h	VAS	IV APAP significantly reduced pain at rest and at 12 hours, nonsignificant reduction in morphine consumption
Total abdominal hysterectomy[4]	Hospitalized women	1 g IV APAP vs PBO	General	Given once either 30 min before surgery or prior to skin closure	VAS	Preemptive IV APAP significantly reduced postop morphine consumption, no hemodynamic effects

Key: APAP, acetaminophen; PBO, placebo; PROP, proparacetamol; VAS, visual analogue scale; VRS, visual rating scale.

[1] Sinatra RS, et al. *Anesthesiology*. 2005;102(4):822-831.

[2] Atef A, Fawaz AA. *Eur Arch Otorhinolaryngol*. 2008;265(3):351-355.

[3] Cattabriga I, et al. *Eur J Cardiothorac Surg*. 2007;32(3):527-531.

[4] Arici S, et al. *Agri*. 2009;21(2):54-61.

In pivotal clinical trials involving >400 patients treated with multiple doses of IV-acetaminophen, elevations twice the upper limit of normal in key liver enzymes ALT and AST were infrequent and equivalent to that observed in patients treated with placebo.[13,15,16] Singla and coworkers[20] evaluated the safety of IV-acetaminophen vs standard analgesic care in >200 patients. They found a numerically lower proportion of patients with elevated liver function tests in the IV-acetaminophen group compared with standard of care. The safety and tolerability of IV-acetaminophen (up to 15 mg/kg) were also tested in 175 pediatric patients requiring analgesic and antipyretic therapy.[21] They found that IV-acetaminophen was well tolerated in this relatively complicated pediatric population, and no clinically relevant differences, severe, or overall treatment-emergent adverse events were noted.

Acetaminophen-induced hepatotoxicity is not caused by the drug itself but from its metabolite NAPQI. Normally, NAPQI undergoes conjugation with glutathione, but at toxic doses glutathione is markedly depleted. Acetaminophen doses exceeding the recommended daily limit and potential toxicity can be treated with *N*-acetylcysteine. *N*-acetylcysteine is a precursor of glutathione and increases the availability of glutathione for NAPQI metabolism. It is most effective if given within 8 to 10 hours of acetaminophen ingestion.[9]

Conclusion

The development and availability of IV-acetaminophen offers the surgeon a new therapeutic option for postsurgical pain management. It offers benefits of:

- High patient safety
- Rapid onset
- Improved analgesic when compared with traditional routes of acetaminophen administration.

For many day-surgical procedures, IV-acetaminophen monotherapy will provide sufficient relief for many of those with mild-to-moderate pain.[22] This can obviate the need or minimize opioid dosing and associated adverse events. When employed in multimodal regimens that involve neural or epidural blockade, IV-acetaminophen can be used for breakthrough pain relief, once again obviating the need for opioid analgesics. When employed with adjunctive IV-PCA or IV opioids, IV-acetaminophen offers benefits of further reductions in pain intensity scores and total opioid dose requirement.[15,23] Despite demonstrated improvements in pain scores, opioid dose, and overall patient satisfaction, studies to date have not been powered to detect significant reductions in opioid-related adverse effects or improvements in postsurgical outcome. In addition, there is an added cost of IV-acetaminophen vs PO and rectal acetaminophen. Additional phase 4 evaluations may demonstrate important pharmacoeconomic benefits associated with IV-acetaminophen treatment and to satisfy pharmacist and administrator concerns regarding increased drug acquisition costs.

REFERENCES

1. Acetaminophen. In: McEvoy GK, ed. *AHFS Drug Information 2003*. McEvoy GK, ed. Acetaminophen. Bethesda, MD: American Society of Health-System Pharmacists; 2003:2077-2085.
2. Anderson BJ. Paracetamol (acetaminophen): mechanisms of action. *Paediatr Anaesth*. 2008;18(10):915-921.
3. Toms L, McQuay HJ, Derry S, Moore RA. Single dose oral paracetamol (acetaminophen) for postoperative pain in adults. *Cochrane Database Syst Rev*. 2008;(4):CD004602.
4. Remy C, Marret E, Bonnet F. State of the art of paracetamol in acute pain therapy. *Curr Opin Anaesthesiol*. 2006;19(5):562-565.
5. Bertolini A, Ferrari A, Ottani A, Guerzoni S. Tacchi R, Leone S. Paracetamol: new vistas of an old drug. *CNS Drug Rev.* 2006; 12(3-4):250-275.
6. Korpela R, Korvenoja P, Meretoja OA. Morphine-sparing effect of acetaminophen in pediatric day-case surgery. *Anesthesiology*. 1999;91(2):442-447.
7. Elia N, Lysakowski C, Tramèr MR. Does multimodal analgesia with acetaminophen, nonsteroidal antiinflammatory drugs, or selective cyclooxygenase-2 inhibitors and patient-controlled analgesia morphine offer advantages over morphine alone? Meta-analyses of randomized trials. *Anesthesiology*. 2005;103(6):1296-1304.
8. Duggan ST, Scott LJ. Intravenous paracetamol (acetaminophen). *Drugs*. 2009;69(1):101-113.
9. Jahr JS, Donkor KN, Sinatra RS. Nonselective nonsteroidal anti-inflammatory drugs, COX-2 inhibitors, and acetaminophen in acute perioperative pain. In: Sinatra RS, de Leon-Cassasola OA, Viscusi ER, Ginsberg B, McQuay H, eds. *Acute Pain Management*. New York, NY: Cambridge University Press; 2009:332-365.
10. Göröcs TS, Lambert M, Rinne T, Krekler M, Modell S. Efficacy and tolerability of ready-to-use intravenous paracetamol solution as monotherapy or as an adjunct analgesic therapy for postoperative pain in patients undergoing elective ambulatory surgery: open, prospective study. *Int J Clin Pract*. 2009;63(1): 112-120
11. Intravenous Acetaminophen (Ofirmev) [package insert]. San Diego, CA: Cadence Pharmaceuticals; 2010.

12. Liukas A, Kuusniemi K, Aantaa R, et al. Pharmacokinetics of intravenous paracetamol in elderly patients. *Clin Pharmacokinet*. 2011;50(2):121-129.

13. Data on file for Ofirmev. San Diego, CA: Cadence Pharmaceuticals; 2010.

14. Royal MA, et al. IV Acetaminophen Administered to Treat Postoperative Pain Significantly Decreases the Incidence of Patient Reporting of Postoperative Fever. Abstract presented at: 2009 Annual Meeting of the American Society of Regional Anesthesia and Pain Medicine; November 19-22, 2009; San Antonio, TX.

15. Sinatra RS, Jahr JS, Reynolds LW, Viscusi ER, Groudine SB, Payen-Champenois C. Efficacy and safety of single and repeated administration of 1 gram intravenous acetaminophen injection (paracetamol) for pain management after major orthopedic surgery. *Anesthesiology*. 2005;102(4):822-831.

16. Miller H, Minkowitz H, Wininger S, Royal M, Breitmeyer J. A phase III, multi-center, randomized, double-blind, placebo-controlled 24 hour study of the efficacy and safety of intravenous acetaminophen in abdominal laparoscopic surgery. Proceedings and Abstracts of the 34th Annual Regional Anesthesia Meeting and Workshops; April 30 to May 3, 2009; Phoenix, AZ. Poster 97.

17. Arici S, Gurbet A, Türker G, Yavaşcaoğlu B, Sahin S. Preemptive analgesic effects of intravenous paracetamol in total abdominal hysterectomy. *Agri*. 2009;21(2):54-61.

18. Breitmeyer JB, Smith HD, Sweeney K, Royal MA. CSF Penetration of Acetaminophen is an Important Determinant of Efficacy. Presented at: 2009 Annual Meeting of the American Society of Regional Anesthesia and Pain Medicine; November 19-22, 2009; San Antonio, TX. Abstract ID: 4.

19. Rømsing J, Møiniche S, Dahl JB. Rectal and parenteral paracetamol, and paracetamol in combination with NSAIDs, for postoperative analgesia. *Br J Anaesth*. 2002;88(2):215-226.

20. Singla N, Ferber L, Bergese S, Royal M, Breitmeyer J. A phase III, multi-center, open-label, prospective, repeated dose, randomized, controlled, multi-day study of the safety of intravenous acetaminophen in adult inpatients. Proceedings and Abstracts of the 34th Annual Regional Anesthesia Meeting and Workshops; April 30 to May 3, 2009; Phoenix, AZ. Poster 96.

21. Krane E, Malviya S, Del Pizzo K, Finkel J, Royal M. Pediatric safety of repeated doses of intravenous acetaminophen. Proceedings and Abstracts of the 34th Annual Regional Anesthesia Meeting and Workshops; April 30 to May 3, 2009; Phoenix, AZ. Poster 58.

22. Atef A, Fawaz AA. Intravenous paracetamol is highly effective in pain treatment after tonsillectomy in adults. *Eur Arch Otorhinolaryngol*. 2008;265(3):351-355.

23. Cattabriga I, Pacini D, Lamazza G, et al. Intravenous paracetamol as adjunctive treatment for postoperative pain after cardiac surgery: a double blind randomized controlled trial. *Eur J Cardiothorac Surg*. 2007;32(3):527-531.

11 Special Considerations: μ-Opioid Receptor Antagonists

by Sergio W. Larach, MD

Pain is usually produced by tissue trauma. Endogenous substances (endorphins and enkephalins) are released by the CNS in response to pain. Exogenous opioids, naturally occurring and synthetic, bind to the opioid receptor, providing highly selective analgesia. Opiate receptors are also distributed throughout the GI tract and assist in GI motility, secretion, and transportation of electrolytes. Localization of these receptors in the GI tract near interneurons, secretomotor neurons, and the interstitial cells of Cajal—the pacemaker cells for GI motility—aids in carrying out these aforementioned biological functions.[1]

There are four types of opioid receptors:

- μ
- κ
- δ
- σ.

The μ-receptor is the primary receptor targeted for the pharmacologic treatment of pain. μ-receptors mediate supraspinal analgesia, respiratory depression, nausea, vomiting, miosis, and bowel hypomotility and are responsible for the main side effects of opioids.[2] The balance between pain control and restoration of bowel activity has led to the development of drugs that can selectively block the nocive response and maintain the pain relief value.

Alvimopan

Alvimopan is a peripheral μ-opioid receptor blocker and was developed in order to reduce GI-related opioid adverse events. It is largely unable to cross the blood-brain barrier and therefore does not block μ-opioid receptors in the CNS or interfere with centrally mediated opioid analgesia. It works in the stomach and bowel to block the effects of opioids in the GI tract. This helps to keep stomach and bowel muscles moving properly. In the treatment of opioid-naïve patients who underwent surgery and received opioids for acute pain, oral alvimopan (6.0 mg) improved the management of postsurgical ileus (POI) by shortening the time to achieve normal bowel function and, ultimately, hospital stay.[1]

When orally administered, after open abdominal partial small- or large-bowel resection in patients with primary anastomosis, alvimopan shortened the return of bowel function and time to discharge by approximately 1 day without compromising analgesia. Alvimopan-treated patients, on average, would account for approximately $900 less (range, $879–$977) in hospital costs than placebo-treated patients due to earlier discharges (and despite the cost of alvimopan [$558] used in the trials). Alvimopan was not shown to be beneficial on these same outcomes after hysterectomy and has not been studied in other surgical populations.

Alvimopan is generally well tolerated when its duration of use is limited, with the frequency of adverse events being similar to placebo when used postsurgically for 1 week or less. Long-term studies of alvimopan in opioid-induced bowel dysfunction have shown an association with adverse cardiovascular outcomes, neoplasms, and fractures. Because of these concerns, the Entereg Access Support and Education program was developed in order to mitigate these risks and minimize the potential for long-term exposure.

The recommended dosage of alvimopan is 12 mg administered with a sip of water 30 minutes to 5 hours before surgery, followed by 12 mg twice daily beginning the day after surgery for a maximum of 7 days, 15 total doses, or until discharge.[1] The wholesale acquisition cost (WAC) for Entereg (alvimopan) is $62.50 for each 12-mg tablet or $937.50 for the entire 7-day treatment course; therefore, the cost-benefit of utilizing opioid-sparing analgesic strategies instead of alvimopan should be considered.[3] The addition of alvimopan to postsurgical management of GI-related opioid adverse events is recommended as a standing order with the enforcement of the preoperative dosage followed by postsurgical dosage in order to ensure the expected result of accelerated return of bowel activity.

Gum Chewing

Another strategy to decrease the incidence of POI has been the implementation of chewing gum in the early postsurgical period. Chewing gum is thought to activate the cephalic phase of digestion mediated by the vagus nerve. Five randomized, controlled trials compared 158 patients who underwent colorectal resection (78 patients received the addition of gum chewing and 80 had standard postsurgical care). All patients tolerated the gum chewing without any side effects. With combined standard postsurgical care and gum chewing, the patients passed flatus 24.3% earlier and had bowel movement 32.7% earlier. The use of gum chewing in the postsurgical period was considered a safe method to stimulate bowel motility and reduce ileus after colorectal surgery.[4]

In another paper, six trials including 244 patients were analyzed. Time to first flatus was significantly reduced with gum chewing plus standard treatment compared with standard treatment alone. In patients with ileus after colonic surgery, gum chewing in addition to standard treatment significantly reduced the time to first flatus and the time to first passage of feces when compared with standard treatment alone. There was also a trend to reduce the length of hospital stay.

The authors suggest that gum chewing should be added to the standard treatment of patients with ileus.[5] There is a hypothesis stating that sugar-free gums that contain hexitols (sorbitol and xylitol) might have laxative effects, which is also a positive effect on prevention of POD.[6]

Conclusion

Combinations of opioid-sparing strategies with demonstrated effectiveness, such as early feeding, epidural analgesia, use of local anesthetic infiltration, laparoscopic or minimally invasive surgery, and peripherally acting μ-opioid receptor antagonists, may help transform the management of POI into an effective multimodal paradigm that targets the diverse etiologic factors leading to this common clinical problem.[7]

REFERENCES

1. Bream-Rouwenhorst HR, Cantrell MA. Alvimopan for postsurgical ileus. *Am J Health Syst Pharm*. 2009;66(14):1267-1277.
2. Sinatra RS. Opioids and opioid receptors. In: Sinatra RS, Jahr JS, Watkins-Pitchford JM, eds. *The Essence of Analgesia and Analgesics*. Cambridge, NY: Cambridge University Press; 2011:73-81.
3. Barletta JF, Asgeirsson T, El-Badawi KI, Senagore AJ. Introduction of alvimopan into an enhanced recovery protocol for colectomy offers benefit in open but not laparoscopic colectomy. *J Laparoendosc Adv Surg Tech A*. 2011;21(10):887-891.
4. Chan MK, Law WL. Use of chewing gum in reducing postsurgical ileus after elective colorectal resection: a systematic review. *Dis Colon Rectum*. 2007;50(12):2149-2157.
5. Vásquez W, Hernández AV, Garcia-Sabrido JL. Is gum chewing useful for ileus after elective colorectal surgery? A systematic review and meta-analysis of randomized clinical trials. *J Gastrointest Surg*. 2009;13(4):649-656.
6. Tandeter H. Hypothesis: hexitols in chewing gum may play a role in reducing postsurgical ileus. *Med Hypotheses*. 2009;72(1):39-40.
7. Saclarides TJ. Current choices–good or bad–for the proactive management of postsurgical ileus: A surgeon's view. *J Perianesth Nurs*. 2006;21(2A suppl):S7-S15.

12

New and Emerging Local Analgesics

by Sonia Ramamoorthy, MD
and Tim Furnish, MD

EXPAREL (bupivacaine liposome injectable suspension)

EXPAREL (bupivacaine liposome injectable suspension) was approved by the FDA in October 2011 and is a liposome injection of bupivacaine, an amide local anesthetic, indicated for single-dose infiltration into the surgical site to produce postsurgical analgesia.[1] In a pivotal trial conducted in a soft tissue surgical model, EXPAREL (bupivacaine liposome injectable suspension) provided postsurgical pain control with reduced opioid requirements for up to 72 hours. EXPAREL (bupivacaine liposome injectable suspension) is bupivacaine encapsulated in a proprietary DepoFoam delivery technology. Two other available products (DepoCyt and DepoDur) use the same DepoFoam technology. Bupivacaine is a well-characterized anesthetic/analgesic with an established safety profile and over 20 years of use in the United States.

DepoFoam is composed of multivesicular liposomes that encapsulate drugs and release them over time. In EXPAREL (bupivacaine liposome injectable suspension), bupivacaine is released from DepoFoam over 96 hours, with the rate of drug delivery partially dependent on the lipid environment. EXPAREL (bupivacaine liposome injectable suspension) is infiltrated locally into the surgical site at the end of surgery using the same technique as developed for standard local anesthetics, including bupivacaine. EXPAREL (bupivacaine liposome injectable suspension) can be administered into the surgical site either undiluted or diluted up to 0.89 mg/mL (ie, 1:14 dilution by volume) with preservative-free normal (0.9%) sterile saline for injection.

EXPAREL (bupivacaine liposome injectable suspension) can easily be administered with a 25-gauge or larger bore needle. EXPAREL (bupivacaine liposome injectable suspension) provides continuous and extended postsurgical analgesia for up to 72 hours.[1] The pharmacokinetics of EXPAREL (bupivacaine liposome injectable suspension) are shown in **Figure 12.1**. The ability to provide postsurgical pain control with

FIGURE 12.1 — EXPAREL (bupivacaine liposome injectable suspension) Plasma Bupivacaine Concentrations (ng/mL) Over Time Following a Single 266-mg Administration

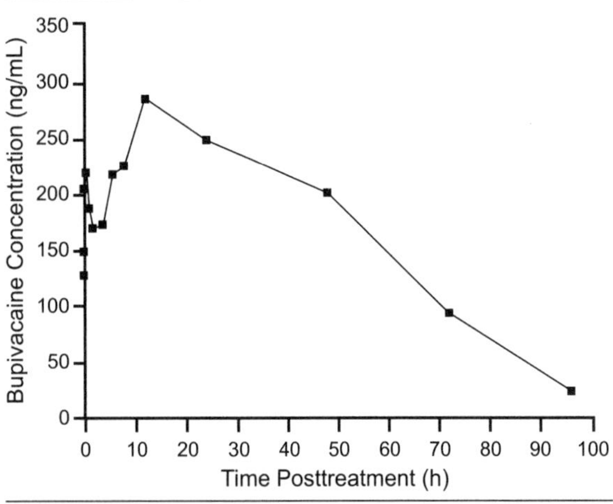

A single, 266-mg intraoperative administration of EXPAREL (bupivacaine liposome injectable suspension) resulted in sustained plasma bupivacaine concentrations (>100 ng/mL) in subjects undergoing inguinal hernia repair.

Langford RM, et al. Poster presented at: 62nd Postgraduate Assembly of the New York State Society of Anesthesiologists; December 12-16, 2008; New York, NY. Poster P-9088.

reduced opioid requirements via a single intraoperative injection results in a significant improvement in their utility to control pain in the postsurgical setting.

The safety of EXPAREL (bupivacaine liposome injectable suspension) injected locally into the surgical site has been evaluated in 10 randomized, double-blind, clinical studies involving 823 patients undergoing various surgical procedures. **Table 12.1** summarizes treatment-emergent adverse reactions with an incidence ≥5% in two placebo-controlled studies. Based on clinical trial data from five active-control, double-blind, randomized trials involving >700 patients undergoing hemorrhoidectomy, total knee arthroplasty, and hernia repair, EXPAREL (bupivacaine liposome injectable suspension) was found to be efficacious in prolonging the time to first narcotic use and reducing overall narcotic use (**Table 12.2**).[2]

In a pivotal phase 3 multicenter, double-blind, randomized, placebo-controlled trial of 189 adults undergoing two- or three-column excisional hemorrhoidectomy, those patients who received a single dose of 1.3%, 20 mL EXPAREL (bupivacaine liposome injectable suspension) experienced a statistically significant 30% reduction in cumulative pain scores (P<0.0001) at 72 hours and at all time points up to 72 hours. The study revealed a statistically significant reduction in the total consumption of opioid rescue medication and a delay in median time to first opioid use compared with placebo (14.3 hours for the EXPAREL (bupivacaine liposome injectable suspension) group vs 1.2 hour for the control group).[3] In a phase 2 trial, EXPAREL (bupivacaine liposome injectable suspension) demonstrated a reduction in pain by 47%, a 66% decrease in opioid use, and reduction in opioid-related adverse events by 89% over standard-dose bupivacaine (75 mg).[1]

The safety of EXPAREL (bupivacaine liposome injectable suspension) has been demonstrated in 21 clinical trials (nine phase 1, seven phase 2, and five phase 3 trials)[4] The most common adverse reactions (incidence ≥10%) following EXPAREL (bupivacaine

TABLE 12.1 — EXPAREL Treatment-Emergent Adverse Events With an Incidence ≥5%: Placebo-Controlled Studies

	Bunionectomy		Hemorrhoidectomy	
System Organ Class ***Preferred Term***	**EXPAREL 106 mg (*N*=97) *n* (%)**	**Placebo (*N*=96) *n* (%)**	**EXPAREL 266 mg (*N*=95) *n* (%)**	**Placebo (*N*=94) *n* (%)**
Any treatment-emergent adverse event	42 (43.3)	38 (39.6)	2 (2.1)	4 (4.3)
Gastrointestinal disorders	40 (41.2)	37 (38.5)	2 (2.1)	4 (4.3)
Nausea	39 (40.2)	36 (37.5)	2 (2.1)	1 (1.1)
Vomiting	27 (27.8)	17 (17.7)	2 (2.1)	4 (4.3)
Nervous system disorders	5 (5.2)	1 (1.0)	0 (0.0)	0 (0.0)
Somnolence	5 (5.2)	1 (1.0)	0 (0.0)	0 (0.0)

TABLE 12.2 — Pooled Analysis of Five Randomized Controlled Trials of EXPAREL vs Bupivacaine

	Exparel (75-300 mg)	Bupivacaine HCl (75-200 mg)	*P* Value
Pain score AUC 0-72 hr	315	427	$P<0.0001$
Median time to first opioid	9.9 hours	2.7 hours	$P<0.0001$
Morphine-equivalent opioid dose	7.9 mg	15.8 mg	$P<0.0001$
Opioid-related adverse events per patient	0.25	0.46	$P<0.0001$

Dasta JF, et al. Presented at: 2011 American College of Clinical Pharmacy Annual Meeting. October 16-19.2011; Pittsburgh, PA. Abstract.

extended-release liposome injection) administration are nausea, constipation, and vomiting. EXPAREL (bupivacaine extended-release liposome injection) did not demonstrate a detectable cardiac toxicity, even at supratherapeutic doses.[5] Furthermore, EXPAREL (bupivacaine liposome injectable suspension) does not require a dose adjustment in patients with mild to moderate hepatic impairment.[1] Importantly, non–bupivacaine-based local anesthetics, including lidocaine, may cause an immediate release of bupivacaine from EXPAREL (bupivacaine liposome injectable suspension) if administered together locally, therefore the administration of EXPAREL (bupivacaine liposome injectable suspension) should not be admixed with lidocaine or other non–bupivacaine-based local anesthetics. That said, EXPAREL (bupivacaine liposome injectable suspension) may be administered after at least 20 minutes or more have elapsed following local administration of lidocaine.

EXPAREL (bupivacaine liposome injectable suspension) has the potential to address a significant unmet medical need for a nonopioid postsurgical analgesic that reduces opioid requirements in the postsurgical setting. This is of particular interest as postsurgical narcotic use is thought to prolong hospitalization by contributing to altered mental status, delayed GI recovery, urinary retention, respiratory depression, and opioid-related adverse events.

Posidur

Another long-acting bupivacaine, SABER-bupivacaine (Posidur), is currently in development. Unlike EXPAREL (bupivacaine liposome injectable suspension), Posidur is a semiviscous gel of sucrose acetate isobutyrate formulation containing 12% bupivacaine that is instilled through a catheter, not injected, into the wound bed. The drug to be delivered by the SABER Delivery System is dissolved or dispersed in a SABER system for instillation. Upon instillation, the

SABER system forms a gel depot from which the drug is delivered at a controlled rate over a period of a few days to 3 months or more.[6,7] Posidur is a sustained-release delivery system using the SABER system to deliver bupivacaine superficially into the wound itself. In a clinical trial using Posidur in postsurgical hernia patients, there was:

- Overall reduction in opioid rescue medication
- Reduced rate of opioid-related side effects
- Improved pain control with movement compared with placebo.[6]

REFERENCES

1. EXPAREL (bupivacaine liposome injectable suspension) [package insert]. San Diego, CA: Pacira Pharmaceuticals, Inc. Web site. http://www.exparel.com/pdf/EXPAREL_Prescribing_Information.pdf. Published November 15, 2011. Accessed December 1, 2011.

2. Dasta JF, Ramamoorthy SL, Patou G, Sinatra R. Bupivacaine extended release liposome injection (DepoFoam bupivacaine) vs bupivacaine HCl: a meta-analysis of multimodal trials of doses up to and including 300 mg. Presented at: 2011 American College of Clinical Pharmacy Annual Meeting; October 16-19, 2011; Pittsburgh, PA. Abstract.

3. Gorfine SR, Onel E, Patou G, Krivokapic ZV. Bupivacaine extended-release liposome injection for prolonged postsurgical analgesia in patients undergoing hemorrhoidectomy: a multicenter, randomized, double-blind, placebo-controlled trial. *Dis Colon Rectum*. 2011;54(12):1552-1559.

4. Bergese SD, Smoot JD, Williams HT. EXPAREL (bupivacaine extended-release liposome injection), an investigational analgesic, provides postsurgical pain relief and decreased opioid use as demonstrated by integrated analysis. Presented at: SAMBA 26th Annual Meeting; May 5, 2011; San Antonio, TX.

5. Naseem A, Harada T, Wang D, et al. Bupivacaine extended release liposome injection does not prolong QTc interval in a thorough QT/QTc study in healthy volunteers [published online ahead of print November 4, 2011]. *J Clin Pharmacol*. doi: 10.1177/0091270011419853.

6. Nicholson D, Brown C, Turner R, et al. Post-operative pain control with extended-release bupivacaine formulation. Clinical trial results in inguinal hernia repair. Presented at: American Hernia Society, 2008 Hernia Repair; March 15, 2008; Scottsdale, AZ. Poster #37. Durect Web site. http://www.durect.com/pdf/Posidur_AHS_2008_Poster.pdf. Accessed November 17, 2011.

7. Post-Operative Pain Depot. Durect Web site. http://www.durect.com/wt/durect/page_name/postop. Accessed December 1, 2011.

13 Postsurgical Pain-Management Strategies in Anorectal Surgery

by Sonia L. Ramamoorthy, MD and Tim Furnish, MD

Introduction

One of the major challenges in managing anorectal pathology is controlling pain and discomfort. Examples of common anorectal pathology include:

- Hemorrhoidal disease
- Anal fissures
- Anal fistula
- Anal pain of unknown etiology (proctalgia fugax).

Most patients have exhausted over-the-counter remedies by the time they are referred for surgical care. Many will never require an operation but instead only require symptomatic relief until the process resolves. Conservative measures for symptomatic relief include:

- Warm tub baths (sitz baths)
- Oral anti-inflammatories by mouth or applied topically
- Stool softeners to reduce trauma to the inflamed area.

Failing these remedies and other targeted therapies, patients are often then referred for surgical intervention.

Local Anesthesia/Analgesia and Anorectal Surgery

Local Anesthesia/Analgesia

Almost all kinds of *simple* anorectal procedures (eg, hemorrhoid banding, proctosigmoidoscopy, skin tag removal, infrared coagulation, etc) are suitable candidates for local anesthetic with or without sedation. The use of local anesthetic alone provides an opportunity for simple procedures to be performed in the office setting. Infiltration with local anesthetic requires knowledge of mechanism of action, duration of action, and infiltration techniques to obtain the maximum benefit for patients and clinicians.

Local anesthetics exert their primary pharmacologic action by inhibiting the excitatory process in nerve endings or nerve fibers. Local anesthetics are broadly classified as either amide or ester, based on the nature of the aromatic linkage between the lipophilic aromatic ring and the hydrophilic amine.[1] The difference between ester and amide anesthetics is in the metabolism and resulting metabolites. Ester local anesthetics have a higher incidence of allergic reactions due to the metabolite paraaminobenzoic acid. Major differences exist in the duration of action of available local anesthetics. Tetracaine spinals will produce a longer-duration block, from 120 to 360 minutes. Procaine spinals will produce a shorter-duration block, from 30 to 60 minutes. A single intraoperative infiltration of EXPAREL (bupivacaine liposome injectable suspension) provides analgesia for up to 72 hours. Dosing for local anesthetics is based on the area to be infiltrated and the particular agent to be used, which is often a weight-based regimen.

Table 13.1 shows various local anesthetics that are used in outpatient and clinical office settings. The most commonly used local anesthetics are lidocaine and bupivacaine, or a mixture of the two, with or without epinephrine. The addition of epinephrine is thought to prolong anesthetic drug effect and assist with hemostasis. Many studies have found this type of anesthesia suitable for simple anorectal procedures.

Lidocaine

Lidocaine is the most common local anesthetic. It can be delivered via local infiltration or as a topical medication. It is most effective for anorectal surgery when infiltrated into the wound bed prior to incision.

Injectable lidocaine comes in various potencies, with or without epinephrine. Lidocaine is available in solutions ranging from 0.5% to 4%, although no studies have compared the efficacy of the different solutions. Lidocaine at 2% concentration may be particularly useful when a smaller injected volume is indicated.[2]

Bupivacaine

Bupivacaine provides an intermediate onset and a longer duration of action. It is especially useful when prolonged anesthesia is needed. Other anesthetics in the amide group can be used in the office but are commonly reserved for spinal and regional anesthesia. Bupivacaine can be administered concomitantly with lidocaine to obtain both rapid-onset anesthetic effect for acute surgical pain and prolonged postsurgical analgesia. Bupivacaine can be administered in variable doses, with common dosing regimens listed in **Table 13.1**.

EXPAREL (bupivacaine liposome injectable suspension)

EXPAREL (bupivacaine liposome injectable suspension) is a nonopioid local analgesic that was recently approved by the FDA for administration into the surgical site to produce postsurgical analgesia. EXPAREL combines bupivacaine with DepoFoam®, a proven product delivery technology that delivers medication over a desired time period. Bupivacaine is present at a concentration of 13.3 mg/mL. After injection of EXPAREL (bupivacaine liposome injectable

TABLE 13.1 — Injectable Local Anesthetics: Pharmacokinetics and Maximal Dose

Anesthetic (Trade) Name	Equivalent Concentration (%)	Onset (min)	Duration (h)	Maximal Dose (mg/kg)	Maximal Dose (mL/70 kg)
Moderate Duration					
Lidocaine (Xylocaine)	1 or 2	<2	1.5 to 2	4 mg/kg, not to exceed 280 mg	28 mL (1%); 14 mL (2%)
Mepivacaine (Carbocaine)	1	3 to 5	0.75 to 1.5	4 mg/kg, not to exceed 280 mg	28 mL
Prilocaine (Citanest)	1	<2	>1	7 mg/kg, not to exceed 500 mg	50 mL
Long Duration					
Lidocaine with epinephrine (Xylocaine injectable)	1 or 2 lidocaine, 1:100,000 or 1:200,000 epinephrine	<2	2 to 6	7 mg/kg, not to exceed 500 mg	Based on lidocaine 50 mL (1%); 25 mL (2%)
Bupivacaine (Marcaine)	0.25	5	2 to 4	2.5 mg/kg, not to exceed 175 mg	50 mL
Etidocaine (Duranest)	0.5 to 1		2 to 3	4 mg/kg, not to exceed 300 mg	50 mL (0.5%)

Very Long Duration				
Bupivacaine liposome injectable suspension (EXPAREL)	1.3%, not bioequivalent to other bupivacaine formulations	5	72	1.3% (13.3 mg/mL), not to exceed 266 mg per surgical site; safety data up to 532 mg

suspension) into soft tissue, bupivacaine is released from the DepoFoam over a period of time. It is indicated for single-dose infiltration into the surgical site to produce postsurgical analgesia. Local infiltration of EXPAREL (bupivacaine liposome injectable suspension) results in significant systemic plasma levels of bupivacaine, which can persist for 96 hours. The efficacy of EXPAREL (bupivacaine liposome injectable suspension) was compared with placebo in two multicenter, randomized, double-blind clinical trials.

One trial evaluated the safety and efficacy of 266 mg EXPAREL (bupivacaine liposome injectable suspension) in 189 patients undergoing hemorrhoidectomy.[3] The mean age was 48 years (range 18 to 86). Study medication was administered directly into the wound (≥3 cm in cumulative wound length) at the conclusion of the surgery. Pain intensity was rated by the patients on a 0 to 10 NRS at multiple time points up to 72 hours. Postsurgically, patients were allowed rescue medication (morphine sulfate 10 mg IM every 4 hours as needed). The primary outcome measure was the AUC of the NRS pain intensity scores (cumulative pain scores) collected over the first 72-hour period. There was a significant treatment effect for EXPAREL (bupivacaine liposome injectable suspension) compared with placebo. In this clinical study, EXPAREL (bupivacaine liposome injectable suspension) demonstrated a significant reduction in pain intensity compared with placebo for up to 24 hours. Between 24 and 72 hours after study drug administration, there was an attendant decrease in opioid consumption.

EXPAREL (bupivacaine liposome injectable suspension) has shown improved patient outcomes with reduced need for postsurgical narcotics and an attendant reduction in narcotic-related adverse events.[4]

■ Techniques for Local Analgesic Infiltration

Local anesthetics can be used in various ways to obtain intraoperative pain relief. Most surgeons prefer to use local anesthetics to create an "anal block" by infiltrating into the intersphincteric groove circumferentially. This can be accomplished in many ways but the use of the "4- or 8-quadrant rule" will ensure adequate anesthesia (**Figure 13.1**). Local infiltration into the specific area of incision (eg, hemorrhoid quadrant, fistula site) is required to ensure adequate anesthesia during the case. Additionally, when performing procedures such as endoanal advancement flap or hemorrhoidectomy, local anesthetics combined with epinephrine are used to "lift mucosal/submucosal flaps" and reduce bleeding at the site.

FIGURE 13.1 — 8-Quadrant Anal Block

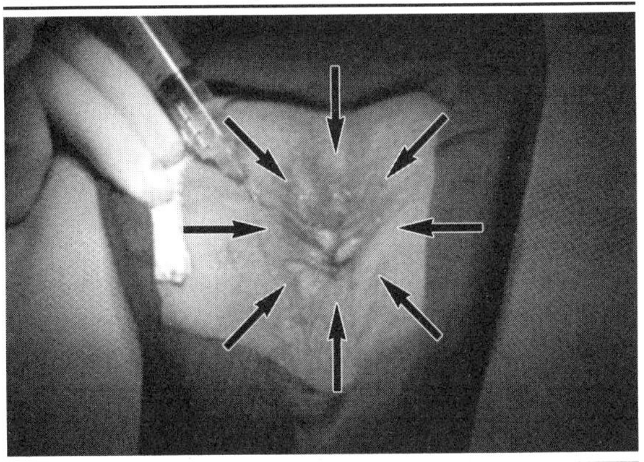

■ Monitored Anesthesia Care (MAC)

The addition of sedation provides the patient added comfort and reduced anxiety, both of which are conducive to a more thorough examination. Moderate sedation requires monitoring and may therefore require an outpatient or hospital setting to administer. Deep sedation, such as with propofol, ketamine, or larger doses of IV sedatives and narcotics, requires the presence of an anesthesiologist for airway protection.

Deep sedation is often used for more invasive procedures, such as excisional hemorrhoidectomy, fistulotomy, or transanal excision. In a randomized study looking at cost and patient outcomes for outpatient anorectal surgery, Li and colleagues found MAC anesthesia to be associated with the highest patient satisfaction, early discharge, and lower costs.[5]

■ Saddle Block and Spinal Analgesia

Spinal local anesthetic analgesia has been in use since the early 20th century. It has a number of clinical advantages, including profound analgesia and motor block without sedation or significant respiratory compromise. Many anorectal procedures are performed using a "spinal" or "saddle block." The term "saddle block" refers to a spinal performed in the sitting position with hyperbaric local anesthetic that then pools around the lumbar and sacral nerve roots. In a recent meta-analysis comparing paravertebral blocks (PVBs) with general anesthesia, PVBs were associated with:

- Shorter LOS
- Improved postsurgical pain control for up to 6 hours postsurgically
- Reduction in postsurgical nausea and vomiting.[6]

Baricity of local anesthetic and patient positioning are the two most important factors in determining the height of the block. The local anesthetic chosen, followed by total dose administered, is the most important factor in determining duration of a spinal anesthetic.

Baricity of local anesthetics is compared with the density of CSF. Hypobaric local anesthetics are less dense than CSF and tend to rise within the intrathecal space relative to patient position, while hyperbaric solutions are denser and will fall within the intrathecal space. Hypobaric solutions are formulated in dextrose and used in saddle blocks for perineal and perianal surgery performed in the lithotomy position. For anorectal surgery performed in the prone jackknife position with head down, a hypobaric spinal can be performed for saddle block. The patient may need to recover in the PACU in a head-down position to prevent cephalad spread of the local anesthetic.

By far the most commonly used local anesthetic for spinal anesthesia is bupivacaine. It is an amide local anesthetic available in hyperbaric and plain isobaric formulations. There are no commercial formulations of hypobaric local anesthetics. Hyperbaric bupivacaine will produce a dense motor and sensory block, lasting from 60 to 240 minutes, depending on dose, patient position, and location of surgery.

Lidocaine spinals have fallen out of favor with many anesthesiologists due to the potential risk of a syndrome known as transient neurologic symptoms (TNS). This manifests as low back, buttock, and posterior thigh pain appearing 6 to 36 hours after recovery from a spinal anesthetic. There are no associated sensory or motor deficits, and patients recover fully within 1 to 7 days. The incidence of TNS is much higher with use of lidocaine and with surgery in the lithotomy position.

Contraindications for spinal and/or saddle block anesthesia include a history of migraines (relative contraindication), the need for perioperative anticoagulation, and previous lower back surgery. Additionally, when compared with MAC anesthesia, spinals are associated with increased rate of urinary retention and longer recovery room stays.[7]

Postsurgical Pain Control in Anorectal Surgery

A recent study reported that the most important predictors of postsurgical pain after ambulatory surgery are:

- Presence of preoperative pain
- Patient and physician expectations regarding the level of pain after the operation
- Patient fear regarding the short-term outcome of their surgery
- Age of the patient.[7]

Postsurgical pain from anorectal surgery is notoriously difficult to control due to the inability to "rest" the area of surgical intervention. Uncontrolled pain, and need for opioid analgesics, can lead to significant morbidity such as urinary retention, constipation, respiratory depression, and other opioid-related complications, as well as added health care expenditures with loss of patient's wages, emergency room visits, and additional medications. Unplanned readmissions after anorectal surgery have been reported to be as high as 17%.[8] Obtaining a balance of adequate pain control that provides comfortable mobility, and bowel and urinary function, while at the same time preventing opioid-related side effects, such as constipation, nausea/vomiting, urinary retention and altered mental status, remains a challenge for most clinicians. The occurrence of a single opioid ADE in hospitalized patients undergoing common surgical procedures has been shown to increase the risk of 30-day readmission by up to 25%. Not only does risk for readmission occur, but increases in risk for LOS and total hospital costs associated with the primary surgical stay increases by 36% and 114%, respectively.[9]

The process begins with a candid discussion with the patient about postsurgical pain and strategies to control it. Applying the concepts of multimodal analgesia has the potential to improve outcomes from anorectal surgery.[3] **Figure 13.2** describes our approach to multimodal analgesia for outpatient anorectal surgery. In these cases, multimodal analgesia benefits the patient by applying multiple layers of pain control, targeting pain relief from several different approaches, while offering the clinician multiple options depending on each patient's specific needs.

One important aspect of multimodal analgesia is the intraoperative administration of local analgesics, such as depo forms of bupivacaine (EXPAREL [bupivacaine liposome injectable suspension]). Local anesthetics are of particular interest as these medications are easily delivered while the patient is still under anesthesia and remain effective during the critical postsurgical period (24 to 96 hours postsurgery). Local analgesic medications have low side effect profiles and few contraindications. Additionally, they reduce

FIGURE 13.2 — Postsurgical Pain Management for Outpatient Anorectal Surgery

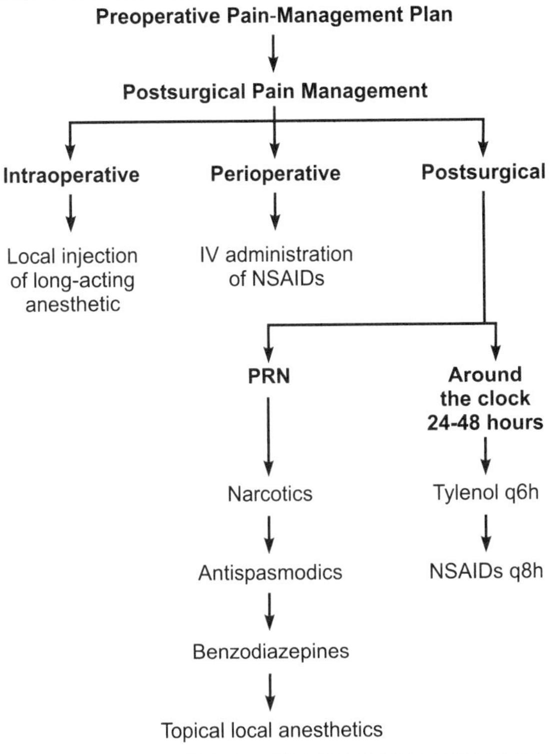

13

the need for postsurgical narcotics, thus expediting functional recovery from anorectal surgery.

It should be noted that in the case of anorectal surgery, the benefits of multimodal analgesia are 2-fold:

- Improved pain control
- Limited use of narcotics, which can adversely effect bowel function and exacerbate pain related symptoms.

In addition to pain medication, the use of preemptive bowel regimens, such as supplemental fiber, stool softeners, sitz baths, and laxatives, are administered to ameliorate the added discomfort of bowel movements immediately postsurgery.

Beyond the standard time periods for recovery from anorectal surgery, there are a small number of patients who may develop more chronic forms of anorectal pain and neuropathic discomfort. Two of the best ways to reduce these risks are to provide adequate pain control in the immediate postsurgical setting and avoid the risk of the "wind-up" phenomenon in the dorsal horns of the spinal cord. Drugs such as pregabalin and gabapentin may be used to alleviate chronic symptoms. These patients are often best served by consultation with a pain specialist.

REFERENCES

1. Sinatra RS, Viscusi G, DeLeon-Cassasola O, Ginsberg B, eds. *Acute Pain Management*. London, England: Cambridge Press; 2009.
2. Achar S, Kundu S. Principles of office anesthesia: part I. Infiltrative anesthesia. *Am Fam Physician*. 2002;66(1) 91-94.
3. Gorfine SR, Onel E, Patou G, Krivokapic ZV. Bupivacaine extended-release liposome injection for prolonged postsurgical analgesia in patients undergoing hemorrhoidectomy: a multi-center, randomized, double-blind, placebo-controlled trial. *Dis Colon Rectum*. 2011;54(12):1552-1559.
4. Dasta JF, Ramamoorthy SL, Patou G, Sinatra R. Bupivacaine extended release liposome injection (DepoFoam bupivacaine) vs bupivacaine HCl: a meta-analysis of multimodal trials of doses up to and including 300 mg. Presented at: 2011 American College of Clinical Pharmacy Annual Meeting; October 16-19, 2011; Pittsburgh, PA. Abstract.
5. Li S, Coloma M, White PF, et al. Comparison of the costs and recovery profiles of three anesthetic techniques for ambulatory anorectal surgery. *Anesthesiology*. 2000;93(5):1225-1230.
6. Thavaneswaran P, Rudkin GE, Cooter RD, Moyes DG, Perera CL, Maddern GJ. Brief reports: paravertebral block for anesthesia: a systematic review. *Anesth Analg*. 2010;110(6):1740-1744.
7. Gramke HF, de Rijke JM, van Kleef M, et al. Predictive factors of postoperative pain after day-case surgery. *Clin J Pain*. 2009; 25(6):455-460.
8. Chan PY, Lee MP, Cheung HY, Chung CC, Li MK. Unplanned admission after day-case haemorrhoidectomy: a retrospective study. *Asian J Surg*. 2010;33(4):203-207.
9. Oderda GM, Gan TJ, Robinson SB, Johnson B. Opioid-related adverse events increase length of stay and drive up total cost of care in a national database of postsurgical patients. Poster presented at: 46th ASHP Midyear Clinical Meeting and Exhibition; December 4-8, 2011; New Orleans, LA. Poster 3-185.

14

Postsurgical Pain-Management Strategies in Abdominal Surgery

by Sergio W. Larach, MD

Seventy-three million patients undergo surgical procedures each year in the United States. Of these, 80% experience acute postsurgical pain, and approximately 20% experience severe pain.[1] The fear of experiencing postsurgical pain and/or adverse events from opioid pain medications are the two most common concerns of surgical patients.[2] The management of acute postsurgical pain and accompanying opioid-related adverse events is often suboptimal, leading to[3]:

- Delayed recovery
- A prolonged hospital stay
- Increased stress and anxiety
- Increased LOS and cost.

Achieving effective pain management while minimizing opioid-related adverse events should be the primary goal in surgical patient care. It includes providing patients with information and appropriate education preoperatively to reduce patient anxiety and instill realistic expectations.[4] Poor pain control may affect the metabolic response and lead to delayed recovery, with subsequent prolonged hospital stays and increased morbidity. It can also lead to chronic pain syndrome. Postsurgical pain control is essential to avoid unnecessary discomfort and prevent complications. Additionally, from the surgeon's point of view, improving postsurgical pain control decreases the risks associated with opioid overdose and complications from analgesic medication, as well as the number of calls to the surgeon from nurses and concerned family members.

In order to establish an appropriate pain-management plan, patient characteristics should be considered, such as:

- Age
- Gender
- Socioeconomic factors
- Medical comorbidities (eg, diabetes, obesity, and sleep apnea)
- Prior opioid use or opioid tolerance
- Preoperative expectations of pain
- Personality traits.

Knowledge about the procedure and prior surgeries are also factors that will influence the patient's expectations and postsurgical pain experience. It is important to have a list of prior medications that have provided relief and also those that have caused secondary undesired effects. In recent studies, advancing age, male gender, and increased severity of illness and length of hospitalization prior to surgical procedure all add to the risk of a patient experiencing opioid-related adverse events and their associated increases in LOS and cost.[5,6]

The level and type of pain experienced in the postsurgical period are personal and influenced by multiple factors. Documentation may be subjective. It is currently being translated with a visual analogue scale (VAS), with a numeric value given to help guide pain management. In addition to monitoring vital signs, pain level should be documented and reported.

Conventional Open Abdominal Surgery

Conventional open abdominal surgery is still being widely performed. The site of surgery and type of intraoperative trauma, including the orientation and size of the incision, degree of visceral manipulation, and surgical trauma, will impact the level of pain after surgery. For example, vertical incisions tend to be more painful due to involvement of more dermatomes. A surgical approach that allows muscle separation is preferred to muscle division. Both surgical trauma and pain are responsible for increased cortisol, endogenous endorphins, catecholamine, and other stress hormone levels. Tachycardia, hypertension, regional decreases in blood flow, alterations in immune response, hyperglycemia, lipolysis, and a negative nitrogen balance can occur as a result of these and other metabolic changes. In response to pain, the patient decreases mobility and is at an increased risk for reduced cough, atelectasis, pneumonia, increased myocardial oxygen consumption and ischemia, constipation, urinary retention and infection, reduced musculoskeletal mobility, and an increased risk of deep venous thrombosis (DVT). These responses highlight the importance of adequate pain control resulting in improved patient outcomes in the perioperative setting.

Minimally Invasive Surgery

An important step forward in postsurgical pain control was added with the implementation of minimally invasive surgery (eg, laparoscopic/robotic, hand-assisted laparoscopy, single-port laparoscopy surgery, etc). Minimally invasive surgery is an important factor in decreasing the amount of postsurgical pain in abdominal surgeries. Surgery on certain specific body organs is now mainly approached using laparoscopic techniques (eg, cholecystectomy, hysterectomy, and prostatectomy), allowing for a shorter hospital stay primarily by allowing for appropriate postsurgical pain control. Pain related to pneumoperitoneum and the incision sites is common to all laparoscopic procedures. Single abdominal-quadrant pathology also shows decreased amount of postsurgical pain compared with a multiquadrant surgical field. The benefits of minimally invasive surgery are such that online patient information for laparoscopic colon resection and cholecystectomy from the Society of American Gastrointestinal and Endoscopic Surgeons (SAGES), widely available for patients to read, indicates that one of the advantages of laparoscopic surgery is less postsurgical pain. Patients are now more informed and educated, and their expectations should be met when possible.

Furthermore, a recent publication comparing the laparoscopic procedures favors the use of the single-port approach based on the fact that one small incision (4.5 cm) leads to less postsurgical pain. Techniques using additional 5-mm ports can cause an increase in postsurgical pain.[7]

Fast-Track Postsurgical Program

The greater advancement in postsurgical management for open and laparoscopic surgeries has been achieved with the implementation of a fast-track postsurgical program.[8] The basic plan consists of:

- Patient preoperative information and education
- Surgical guidelines for nursing care, including early mobilization
- Early feeding and no use of nasogastric tubes
- Adequate pain control implemented with multimodal therapy to minimize the use of any single analgesic.

Local Analgesics in Abdominal Surgery

One way of reducing somatic pain in abdominal surgery is by using local anesthetics. Abdominal surgery pain tends to be long lasting, so the longer a local anesthetic works, the better for the patient. Local anesthetics can be used through local wound infiltration. Intraincisional infiltration with a bupivacaine/epinephrine mixture significantly reduces abdominal postsurgical pain and narcotic analgesic consumption.[9] Local administration of local anesthetics, including EXPAREL (bupivacaine liposome injectable suspension), has been demonstrated to be safe and effective in hemorrhoidectomy and herniorrhaphy.[10,11] Another approach to control pain is to use shorter-acting local anesthetics through catheters placed in the incision site. However, in a recent meta-analysis review by Gupta and associates, wound catheters provided no significant analgesia at rest or on activity except in patients undergoing gynecologic and obstetric surgery at 48 hours, although the overall morphine consumption in the first 24 hours was lower in these patients.[12]

Another modality of pain control can be established with placement of epidural anesthesia. It is effective for postsurgical pain relief and results in earlier recovery from postsurgical paralytic ileus. Epidural anesthesia use also shows a reduction in respiratory complications such as pneumonia.[13] A study comparing use of thoracic epidural anesthetic (TEA) in patients undergoing laparoscopic colorectal resection (39 in the TEA group and 36 in the non-TEA group) concluded that TEA provides a significant benefit in terms of less analgesic consumption, better postsurgical pain relief, and faster recovery of GI function in patients undergoing such surgery.[14]

The use of both intermediate- and long-acting local anesthetics at laparoscopic port sites through wound infiltration is also part of an effective multimodal analgesic approach. A combination of intraperitoneal, perifascial, and subcutaneous bupivacaine with epinephrine provides significant morphine-sparing analgesia for 4 hours after total abdominal hysterectomy.[15] Continuous paravertebral anesthetics result in improved analgesia and reduced pulmonary complications in nonobese patients.[16]

Patient-Controlled Analgesia (PCA)

Opioid analgesics are the cornerstone for pain control and different routes of administration are useful. In US hospitals, >95% of patients undergoing common surgical procedures are administered opioids during their postsurgical course.[5] As many as 80% experience some sort of opioid-related adverse event.[2] The main side effects of drugs of this class are:

- Respiratory depression
- Nausea
- Vomiting
- Constipation
- Urinary retention
- Physical dependence.

The opioids commonly used for PCA are morphine, hydromorphone, and fentanyl. Standard PCA orders are strongly recommended (**Table 14.1**), such as:

- Morphine: 1 mg to 2 mg, with lockout period of 6 minutes, for a maximum dose of 30 mg in 4 hours.
  - Attention should be placed on drug interactions, such as barbiturates, benzodiazepines, and antihistamines.
  - Common side effects are managed with naloxone, the drug of choice for reversal of respiratory depression.
  - To palliate nausea and vomiting and in addition to opioid-sparing strategies, ondansetron, metoclopramide, droperidol, and steroids are commonly used.
  - Pruritus can be controlled with Benadryl.
  - Urinary retention usually requires the placement of a urinary catheter and often delays discharge.
- Hydromorphone: Dilaudid 0.2 mg to 0.4 mg, with a lockout period of 6 minutes, for a maximum dose of 6 mg in 4 hours.
- Fentanyl: 10 mcg to 20 mcg, with a lockout period of 4 minutes, for a maximum dose of 325 mcg in 4 hours.
  - Fentanyl has drug interactions and side effects similar to those of morphine.

The use of opioid PCA pumps should be limited to the first 24 hours postsurgery whenever possible. Patients

TABLE 14.1 — Standard PCA Orders

Medication	PCA Dose	Lockout Interval	Mandatory 4-Hour Limit
Morphine (30 mg/30 mL)	1-2 mg	6-10 min	Max 30 mg
Hydromorphone (Dilaudid) (6 mg/30 mL)	0.2-0.4 mg	6-10 min	Max 6 mg
Fentanyl (300 mcg/30 mL)	10-20 mcg	4-6 min	Max 325 mcg

should be switched to oral analgesics (opioid and non-opioid) as soon as the patient's progress allows, based on the amount of opioid pump use observed during the prior 24 hours to achieve pain control.

There are many publications in the current literature supporting the use of opioid PCA postsurgery. In a Cochrane database review, 55 studies with 2023 patients receiving PCA and 1838 patients assigned to a control group met inclusion criteria. PCA provided better pain control and greater patient satisfaction than conventional parenteral as-needed analgesia. Patients using PCA consumed higher amounts of opioids than the controls and had a higher incidence of pruritus but had a similar incidence of other adverse effects. There was no difference in the length of hospital stay. This review provides evidence that PCA is an efficacious alternative to conventional, as-needed systemic analgesia for postsurgical pain control.[17]

Oral Multimodal Analgesia

Multimodal analgesia is achieved by combining different analgesics that act by different mechanisms, reducing adverse effects of the sole administration of individual analgesics.[18] Different types of analgesics include opioids (eg, morphine, fentanyl, tramadol, codeine) used with a nonopioid (eg, ketorolac, NSAID, COX-2 inhibitor, acetaminophen), delivered through various routes (**Table 14.2**). Administration of analgesia by local anesthetics (bupivacaine and EXPAREL [bupivacaine liposome injectable suspension]) also decreases pain and the need for narcotic medications by reducing the noxious stimuli produced by tissue injury.

Concomitant to opioid PCA use, IV NSAIDs and/or acetaminophen are commonly used. Orally available agents should be converted to the oral form promptly as the clinical course progresses (**Table 14.3**). Ketorolac (Toradol) dosage is 15 mg to 30 mg IV every 6 hours, not to exceed 5 days of use. Ketorolac dose is adjusted based on age and kidney function, not to exceed 60

TABLE 14.2 — Oral Multimodal Analgesics

Medication	Dose
Tramadol	50-100 mg every 4-6 hours
Oxycodone	5-30 mg every 4-6 hours
Hydrocodone	5-10 mg every 4-6 hours
Ketorolac	10 mg every 6 hours
Ibuprofen	400-800 mg every 8 hours
Diclofenac sodium	25-75 mg every 8 to 12 hours
Celebrex	50-400 mg daily
Acetaminophen	325-650 mg every 4-6 hours

TABLE 14.3 — Intravenous NSAIDs and Acetaminophen

Generic (Trade) Name	Dose
Ketorolac (Toradol)	15-30 mg IV every 6 hours, not to exceed 5 days
Ibuprofen (Caldolor)	400-800 mg IV every 6 hours, not to exceed 3200 mg daily
Acetaminophen (Tylenol)	1 g IV, not to exceed 4 g daily

mg/day in patients >65 year of age, with renal impairment, and <50 kg in body weight. Ibuprofen is also used as multimodal therapy in doses of 400 mg to 800 mg IV every 6 hours, not to exceed 3200 mg in 24 hours. Acetaminophen (Tylenol) dosage is 1 g IV, not to exceed 4 g daily (less in patients at risk for liver damage). The regimens of IV acetaminophen (1000 mg every 6 hours and 650 mg every 4 hours) were associated with statistically significant analgesic efficacy compared with placebo and were well tolerated in adults after abdominal laparoscopic surgery.[19]

It appears that ketorolac provides a better postsurgical course than either IM or PCA morphine in terms of pain control, postsurgical confusion, LOS, and duration of ileus. Most patients should probably be managed with PCA narcotics, but the addition of ketorolac might reduce narcotic dose and resultant adverse effects. Those patients particularly prone to adverse effects should receive ketorolac primarily.[20] The adverse effects to be considered with nonselective NSAIDs include altered platelet aggregation, which should be accounted for in patients with an increased risk of bleeding. COX-2 inhibitors are used to decrease the risk of GI damage.

Oral combination medication of opioid and nonopioid analgesics can be used after the patient resumes oral intake and is discharged home. Oxycodone, hydrocodone, or tramadol, alone or combined with acetaminophen, can be used, not exceeding the maximum doses indicated. Use of oxycodone alone may be advantageous in those patients who are at risk for toxicity from NSAIDs or acetaminophen.

Abdominal Surgery in the Elderly Patient

The elderly abdominal surgery patient presents a special set of challenges due to their diminished tolerance of the side effects caused by opioid and nonopioid analgesic therapy. Dosages and dosing intervals often need to be modified based on the presence of common comorbidities such as renal disease and dementia, as well as concomitant medications (CNS, anticoagulants, etc). The assessment of mental status, bleeding risk, vital signs, level of sedation, and pain score should be frequently performed for optimal pain control in the elderly. It is known that advancing age is a clear risk factor for opioid-related adverse events and, when they occur, they often lead to increased LOS and cost.[5]

In elderly patients with normal mental status, the use of an opioid PCA delivery system is preferred since it may reduce overall opioid consumption, therefore diminishing the chances of opioid-related side effects and improving overall analgesia. Unfortunately, some elderly patients with underlying dementia or postsurgical mental status changes or delirium cannot manage self-administered analgesia through the PCA pump. In these patients, multimodal therapy, including the use of local anesthetics infiltrated locally, will provide a safer and more efficient pain-management plan.

Conclusion

Surgeons need to consider that variables inherent to the patient, such as age, gender, ethnicity, comorbidities, use of prior opioids, socioeconomic status, individual pain threshold, and prior surgical experience, will affect the level of postsurgical pain and response to treatment. A proper medical history, including history of medication use, should be completed to guide adequate pain management postsurgery. The combination of the surgical approach, incision size, and local pain-control modalities, with the use of multimodal opioid and nonopioid combinations including local anesthetic infiltration, will ensure a faster postsurgical recovery and minimize short-term and long-term complications associated with inadequate pain control and the use of opioid therapy (**Figure 14.1**).

FIGURE 14.1 — Pain-Management Planning

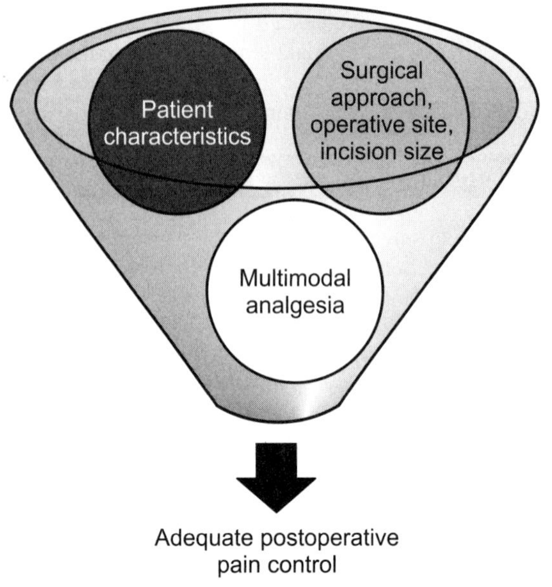

Adequate postoperative pain control

REFERENCES

1. Hutchison RW. Challenges in acute post-operative pain management. *Am J Health Syst Pharm*. 2007;64(6 suppl 4):S2-S5.
2. Gan TJ, Lubarsky DA, Flood EM, et al. Patient preferences for acute pain treatment. *Br J Anaesth*. 2004;92(5):681-688.
3. Harden N, Cohen M. Unmet needs in the management of neuropathic pain. *J Pain Symptom Manage*. 2003;25(5 suppl):S12-S17.
4. Al Samaraee A, Rhind G, Saleh U, Bhattacharya V. Factors contributing to poor post-operative abdominal pain management in adult patients: a review. *Surgeon*. 2010;8(3):151-158.
5. Oderda GM, Gan TJ, Robinson SB, Johnson B. Opioid-related adverse events increase length of stay and drive up total cost of care in a national database of postsurgical patients. Poster presented at: 46th ASHP Midyear Clinical Meeting and Exhibition; December 4-8, 2011; New Orleans, LA. Poster 3-185.
6. Moleski R, Adamson R, Lew I. Cost and quality implications of opioid-based post surgical pain control in total abdominal hysterectomy: a study of cost outliers and opioid related adverse events. Poster presented at: 46th ASHP Midyear Clinical Meeting and Exhibition; December 4-8, 2011; New Orleans, LA. Poster 3-192.
7. Papaconstantinou HT, Sharp N, Thomas JS. Single-incision laparoscopic right colectomy: a case-matched comparison with standard laparoscopic and hand-assisted laparoscopic techniques. *J Am Coll Surg*. 2011;213(1):72-80.
8. Christensen HK, Thaysen HV, Rodt SÅ, Carlsson P, Laurberg S. Short hospital stay and low complication rate are possible with a fully implemented fast-track model after elective colonic surgery. *Eur Surg Res*. 2011;46(3):156-161.
9. Lepner U, Goroshina J, Samarütel J. Postoperative pain relief after laparoscopic cholecystectomy: a randomised prospective double-blind clinical trial. *Scand J Surg*. 2003;92(2):121-124.
10. Gorfine SR, Onel E, Patou G, Krivokapic ZV. Bupivacaine extended-release liposome injection for prolonged postsurgical analgesia in patients undergoing hemorrhoidectomy: a multicenter, randomized, double-blind, placebo-controlled trial. *Dis Colon Rectum*. 2011;54(12):1552-1559.
11. Langford, RM, Chappell GM, Karrasch JA. A single administration of depobupivacaine intraoperatively results in prolonged detectable plasma bupivacaine and analgesia in patients under-

going inguinal hernia repair. Presented at: 62nd Postgraduate Assembly of the New York State Society of Anesthesiologists; December 12-16, 2008; New York, NY. Poster P-9088.

12. Gupta A, Favaios S, Perniola A, Magnuson A, Berggren L. A meta-analysis of the efficacy of wound catheters for post-operative pain management. *Acta Anaesthesiol Scand.* 2011;55(7):785-796.

13. Warschkow R, Steffen T, Lüthi A, et al. Epidural analgesia in open resection of colorectal cancer: is there a clinical benefit? A retrospective study on 1,470 patients. *J Gastrointest Surg.* 2011;15(8):1386-1393.

14. Zingg U, Miskovic D, Hamel CT, Erni L, Oertli D, Metzger U. Influence of thoracic epidural analgesia on postoperative pain relief and ileus after laparoscopic colorectal resection: Benefit with epidural analgesia. *Surg Endosc.* 2009;23(2):276-282.

15. Ng A, Swami A, Smith G, Davidson AC, Emembolu J . The analgesic effects of intraperitoneal and incisional bupivacaine with epinephrine after total abdominal hysterectomy. *Anesth Analg.* 2002;95(1):158-162.

16. Joshi GP, Bonnet F, Shah R, et al. A systematic review of randomized trials evaluating regional techniques for postthoracotomy analgesia. *Anesth Analg.* 2008;107(3):1026-1040.

17. Hudcova J, McNicol E, Quah C, Lau J, Carr DB. Patient controlled opioid analgesia versus conventional opioid analgesia for postoperative pain. *Cochrane Database Syst Rev.* 2006;(4): CD003348.

18. Kehlet H, Dahl JB. The value of "multimodal" or "balanced analgesia" in postoperative pain treatment. *Anesth Analg.* 1993; 77(5):1048-1056.

19. Wininger SJ, Miller H, Minkowitz HS, et al. A randomized, double-blind, placebo-controlled, multicenter, repeat-dose study of two intravenous acetaminophen dosing regimens for the treatment of pain after abdominal laparoscopic surgery. *Clin Ther.* 2010;32(14):2348-2369.

20. Nitschke LF, Schlösser CT, Berg RL, Selthafner JV, Wengert TJ, Avecilla CS. Does patient-controlled analgesia achieve better control of pain and fewer adverse effects than intramuscular analgesia? A prospective randomized trial. *Arch Surg.* 1996;131(4):417-423.

15

Postsurgical Pain-Management Strategies in Special Populations

by Sonia Ramamoorthy, MD, Tim Furnish, MD, Garth Jacobsen, MD, and Alisa Cocker, MD

Certain patient populations in surgery warrant special consideration with regard to postsurgical pain management. In colorectal surgery, those populations most commonly include:

- The obese patient
- The elderly (>75 years of age)
- Opioid-tolerant individuals.

The Obese Patient

Pain is the most frequently encountered postsurgical problem after open or laparoscopic bariatric surgery.[1] In addition to providing patient comfort, adequate analgesia allows for greater patient compliance with early mobilization, reducing the risk of DVT, pressure ulcers, and respiratory complications.[2]

In order to provide adequate analgesia and manage patient expectations, the physician should have an understanding of other medical conditions that may interact with postsurgical pain and how the patient interprets it. Nearly half of all bariatric patients are taking psychotropic medications, and the population has been shown to have a high prevalence of depression, posttraumatic stress disorder (PTSD), and anxiety.[3] A recent study has shown that previous psychiatric hospitalization, unmarried status, younger age, and male gender are associated with greater opioid use following bariatric surgery.[4] In addition, a recent retrospective study in common surgical procedures has identified the elderly, male gender, and increasing severity of illness as significant risk factors to increased LOS and total hospital costs when an opioid-related adverse event occurs postsurgically.[5]

Special consideration should be given to safety and monitoring in the bariatric population. Obstructive sleep apnea (OSA) is common in this population.[6] While OSA as an independent risk factor for pulmonary complications has been widely debated, it is documented that opioid administration enhances OSA in predisposed patients.[7] Considering obese patients have increased desaturation events with or without an OSA diagnosis,[8] the cautious physician will use opioids, which are associated with central apnea, judiciously and in a monitored setting with continuous pulse oximetry, sedation monitoring, and capnography. Note, however, that routine admission of obese patients with OSA to the ICU is not required, as this does not affect pulmonary complication rates or perioperative course.[9]

■ Preoperative Considerations

In addition to managing pain postsurgically, the surgeon should be thinking of what can be done preoperatively and intraoperatively to reduce postsurgical pain. Use of local anesthetics during surgery as part of a multimodal pain regimen has been shown to reduce postsurgical opioid use.[10] Regional anesthetic techniques have the advantage of reducing postsurgical opioid use and thus the associated complications.

One retrospective study of bariatric-surgery patients looked at morphine PCA vs epidural anesthesia that included morphine or fentanyl. There was no difference identified in length of hospital stay, pain control at rest, or pain control at first ambulation. There was a higher incidence of postsurgical nausea and vomiting and later return of bowel function in the morphine PCA group.[11] Criticism of this study included the lack of local anesthetic use in the morphine group and that the thoracic epidurals were inserted at a low level (Th12-

L2).[12] In the nonobese population, standard thoracic epidural analgesia with local anesthetics has beneficial effects on pulmonary function and reduces complications.[7] Assuming the applicability of this effect in the obese population and the potential for superior analgesia with less adverse effects on bowel function, this is a method that should be considered in major bariatric surgery. However, there is conflicting evidence to support routine use, and the cost and potential risks of thoracic epidurals should be considered.

■ Postsurgical Treatment

Given the risk of gastric perforation, nonselective NSAIDs should be used with caution following bariatric surgery.[7] Nevertheless, significant improvement in postsurgical pain control can be obtained with the use of NSAIDs such as ketorolac.[7] If the surgeon has a high concern for postsurgical bleeding, GI complications, or cardiovascular events given the patient's history and comorbidities, a selective coxib, such as celecoxib, could be considered.[7,13] Studies with ibuprofen indicate higher doses with the same dosing frequency may be necessary in the obese population.[14]

Acetaminophen, while shown to be inferior to NSAIDs in multimodal analgesia, should be considered in patients with contraindications to NSAIDs.[15] While studies in rodents have shown an increased risk of liver and kidney damage,[16] this has not been substantiated in human studies.[17] Studies indicate this can be dosed according to ideal weight.[7]

The use of opioids, even with the above-mentioned measures, often cannot be avoided in the postsurgical period. The amount required for adequate analgesia appears to be widely variable according to several studies looking at morphine requirements in obese subjects.[7] Given this, administration of opioids via PCA may provide the best results. PCA administration offers analgesic titratability, which may be beneficial in improving pain and pulmonary function in obese patients.[18-23] A major issue with IV-PCA in morbidly obese patients is the use of basal opioid infusions, which increase the risk of sleep apnea and probably should not be used unless the patients are opioid dependent. Concerns have also been raised about the use of PCA in morbidly obese patients who have obstructive sleep apnea (OSA). A near-fatal case of respiratory depression was reported by VanDercar and colleagues associated with PCA use in a patient with OSA.[23] However, the PCA machine was set to deliver a background infusion, as well as patient-demand doses.

PCA, without a background infusion, has been used safely and effectively for pain relief after abdominal surgery in morbidly obese patients, up to 40% of whom may have OSA. If patients are known to have OSA, more intensive monitoring and judicious use of PCA (eg, use of a smaller initial bolus dose) have been suggested.

The Elderly Patient

Persons over the age of 65 represent the fastest growing population in the United States today, with those over 80 years of age the fastest growing subsection of older persons.[24] As a result, a higher proportion of those presenting for surgery in the future will be older, including greater numbers aged over 100 years. Postsurgical pain management in these patients can be complicated by factors such as age and disease-related changes in physiology, neurocognitive disorders (both diagnosed and undiagnosed), and disease-drug and drug-drug interactions. Age is one of the most commonly overlooked and yet one the most important patient variables influencing analgesic response, sensitivity to opioid-related adverse events and perioperative outcome.

In a study by Monk and colleagues,[25] at the time of discharge, >40% of older patients had postsurgical cognitive dysfunction and 12.7% still suffered the cognitive problems after 3 months. They also found that patients who suffer postsurgical cognitive dysfunction are at increased risk of death within a year of the surgery. Patients with postsurgical cognitive dysfunction at discharge were also more likely than other patients to be taking opioids; the pain medication or persisting postsurgical pain itself may have affected their performance on cognitive testing.

Alterations in pharmacokinetics and pharmacodynamics may influence drugs and techniques used for pain relief. Advancing age can alter analgesic dose response in several ways. A decrease in hepatic enzymes, particularly CYP-450 microsomes and glucuronidases, as well as diminished hepatic blood flow, can reduce opioid and local anesthetic metabolism and delay drug elimination. Age-related reductions in plasma albumin may increase the fraction of unbound or active drug, while diminished pain transmission and CNS activity may significantly reduce perception and subsequent processing of pain.[26] The elderly may also have impaired renal clearance and are more susceptible to toxicities from commonly used postsurgical pain medications such as nonsteroidal agents and meperidine. With appropriate dose/frequency adjustments and close monitoring, these medications can be used safely in an elderly patient.

Close attention should be made to available data provided by manufacturers with regard to the experience of medication use in elderly patients. One example is with the recently approved local analgsic, EXPAREL (bupivacaine liposome injectable suspension), where 171 of the total number of patients in the EXPAREL (bupivacaine liposome injectable suspension) wound infiltration clinical studies (N=823) were ≥65 years of age and 47 patients were ≥75 years of age. No overall differences in safety or effectiveness were observed between these patients and younger patients. The importance for new agents to reduce the amount of opioids required to provide the same, or superior, pain control in our ever-increasing number of elderly patients serves as advancement in postsurgical pain control.[27]

The evidence-base for postsurgical pain management in the older population remains limited. Most commonly used analgesic regimens are suitable for older patients if adapted and titrated appropriately. Many surgeons will anecdotally recognize that the elderly patient requires less postsurgical medication than younger age groups by comparison. In a study by Gagliese and coworkers, it was observed that on the first postsurgical day, young patients consumed an average of 66.6 mg PCA with morphine, whereas older patients consumed an average of only 39.1 mg.[28] Based on these findings, the authors suggested the following formula for determining the average morphine requirement based on patient age:

{Average postsurgical 24-hour morphine use (mg) = 100 – age (years).}

Although less opioid may be required in the elderly, the incidence of opioid-related adverse events after common surgical procedures tends to be higher in the elderly[5] and, when they occur, result in significantly longer LOS and total hospital costs. Intact cognition is essential for optimal use of IV and epidural PCA. Several studies revealed that advancing age is associated with decreased self-administration of opioids,[29] possibly because elderly patients perceive less postsurgical pain and are less willing or less able to use the PCA device. Inadequate analgesia was also previously found to be more frequent among elderly patients, a finding that again may be related to baseline cognitive deficits or acute postsurgical confusional states.[12-15]

Given several confounding variables associated with pain management in the elderly, these patients are best served by multimodal analgesia regimens that engage multiple metabolic pathways. Special consideration should be given to the physiologic and neurocognitive challenges that can impact this age group.

The Opioid-Tolerant Patient

The use of opioids for managing chronic nonmalignant pain and the illicit use of prescription opioids for recreational purposes have increased substantially over the past decade. In the United States, prescription opioids result in two patient deaths per hour and nearly 40 emergency department visits.[30] Patients requiring surgery who are chronic users of opioids pose a special challenge in the management of postsurgical pain. They are at increased risk for severe postsurgical pain and increased opioid-related adverse events, as well as the development of chronic postsurgical pain. The large doses of opioid medications required to control their pain tend to make nurses and physicians uncomfortable, as well as increase their risk of dose-limiting adverse events and, as a result, they may have pain that is undertreated in the postsurgical period. Undertreatment of pain increases the risk of:

- Hypertension
- Tachycardia
- Atelectasis from shallow respiration
- Potentially, impaired wound healing due to elevated catecholamines and hyperglycemia.

Another risk of chronic opioid use is opioid-induced hyperalgesia. This condition may occur in patients who are on high doses of opioids over time. Opioid-induced hyperalgesia results in hypersensitivity to mildly noxious stimuli and pain out of proportion to the injury. The mechanism for opioid-induced hyperalgesia is unknown and there is no clear way of reversing the hypersensitivity. In some clinical models, ketamine infusions under general anesthesia have reduced this hypersensitive state.

There has been increasing evidence regarding the effectiveness of nonopioid analgesics given before and during surgery for reducing pain scores and opioid requirements in the immediate postsurgical period. These analgesics, given preemptively, reduce nociceptive input to, and resulting sensitization of, dorsal horn neurons in the spinal cord. Sensitization of these neurons occurs with surgical stimulus and contributes to a hyperalgesic state postsurgically, with heightened levels of pain in the periincisional noninjured tissue. Patients on chronic opioids are at higher risk for this central sensitization. Nonopioid agents, such as locally administered analgesics, slow sensory input to the dorsal horn neurons and will decrease this sensitization. A one-time dose of gabapentin or pregabalin an hour before surgery reduces pain scores and postsurgical opioid requirements and may decrease chronic pain that can occur weeks to months after surgery. The typical doses given in the preoperative area are 600 to 1200 mg of gabapentin or 150 mg of pregabalin.

Ketamine infusions during surgery have been used with similar analgesic effects. Developed as an IV anesthetic agent for the induction of general anesthesia, ketamine has been in use since the 1960s. It produces a dissociative anesthetic state with amnesia and profound analgesia without causing respiratory depression, nausea, or decreased GI motility. It can cause hallucinations, bad dreams, and increased salivation, but given in a low-dose infusion under general anesthesia, these adverse effects are uncommon or minimal. The efficacy of a low-dose infusion during surgery on reducing postsurgical pain and opioid requirements has been shown for spinal fusions, total abdominal hysterectomy, and other surgical procedures. Typical protocols include an infusion of 5-10 mcg/kg/minute with or without a loading dose of 0.3-0.5 mg/kg. There is some evidence that the effectiveness of ketamine for postsurgical pain management is greater in the opioid-tolerant than in the opioid-naïve patient.

Opioid-tolerant patients will have increased postsurgical opioid requirements compared with the opioid-naïve patient. Some studies have shown that they may need up to three times the opioid doses that a nontolerant patient requires. Special consideration needs to be made in these patients as it relates to opioid-related adverse events; although their analgesic opioid threshold may increase, their threshold to opioid-related adverse events usually does not. Considerations for initial postsurgical management of opioid-tolerant patients are shown in **Table 15.1**.

Additionally, with the recent approval of the local analgesic EXPAREL (bupivacaine liposome injectable suspension), clinicians now have the added benefit of treating incisional pain for up to 3 days with medications other than opioid-based pain medications, which has significant implications in this patient population.

Opioid-tolerant patients undergoing major surgery are much more likely than others to need a consultation with a pain specialist. If the management of their postsurgical pain is challenging, consider nonopioid-based alternatives and calling for a pain consult sooner rather than later or even preoperatively. Expect that the duration of their hospitalization will be longer than typical and may require more intensive multidisciplinary assistance before and after surgery, including anesthesiology, physical therapy, psychology, social work, and pain-management specialists.

TABLE 15.1 — Initial Postsurgical Management of Opioid-Tolerant Patients

- Continue baseline long-acting opioids (eg, fentanyl patch, oxycodone, or sustained-release morphine) to control baseline (presurgical pain) and to prevent withdrawal.
- Multimodal analgesia with agents that work on a variety of receptors is even more important in the opioid tolerant. Using a combination of opioid and nonopioid agents may improve analgesia while reducing opioid doses and adverse effects from use of a single agent. Acetaminophen, NSAIDs, and local analgesics are commonly used nonopioid agents. For patients who are NPO, Toradol (ketorolac) and Ofirmev (acetaminophen) are IV nonopioid options. Infiltration of the wound and surrounding tissues with long-acting local anesthetics can assist with reduction of pain itself and in postsurgical opioid requirements.
- Use PCA or short-acting IV and oral opioids on top of baseline opioid regimen for increased pain from surgery. Starting dose on PCA will likely need to be higher than for a nontolerant patient and may need to be titrated to higher doses if starting dose is ineffective at managing pain.
- To prevent confusion, avoid using multiple short-acting opioids simultaneously.
- Include a nurse-administered IV bolus dose that is two to three times higher than the PCA bolus dose for rescue analgesia. An IV bolus dose is important for control of pain that occurs sporadically with dressing changes, ambulation, and physical therapy or while titrating PCA to an appropriate dose (should be available every 2 to 4 hours initially).
- Patients who are experiencing painful muscle spasm may benefit from the addition of a muscle relaxant, such as cyclobenzaprine, diazepam, or tizanidine, either PRN or scheduled.
- Anxiety combined with postoperative pain will increase distress, and the experience of pain will be heightened. Use of a benzodiazepine may help manage anxiety and distress as well as muscle spasm.
- Use of neuraxial analgesia (eg, spinal or epidural) during and after surgery will decrease the supplemental opioid requirements and improve postoperative pain. Epidural analgesia with local anesthetics also results in abdominal vasodilatation with more rapid return of GI function.

REFERENCES

1. Leykin Y, Pellis T, Del Mestro E, Fanti G, Marzano B. Perioperative management of 195 consecutive bariatric patients. *Eur J Anaesthesiol*. 2008;25(2):168-170.
2. Kaffarnik M, Utzolino S. [Postoperative management of patients with BMI > 40 kg / m2]. *Zentralbl Chir*. 2009;134(1): 43-49. German.
3. Pawlow LA, O'Neil PM, White MA, Byrne TK. Findings and outcomes of psychological evaluations of gastric bypass applicants. *Surg Obes Relat Dis*. 2005;1(6):523-527; discussion 528-529.
4. Weingarten TN, Sprung J, Flores A, Baena AM, Schroeder DR, Warner DO. Opioid requirements after laparoscopic bariatric surgery. *Obes Surg*. 2011;21(9):1407-1412.
5. Oderda GM, Gan TJ, Robinson SB, Johnson B. Opioid-related adverse events increase length of stay and drive up total cost of care in a national database of postsurgical patients. Poster presented at: 46th ASHP Midyear Clinical Meeting and Exhibition; December 4-8, 2011; New Orleans, LA. Poster 3-185.
6. Frey WC, Pilcher J. Obstructive sleep-related breathing disorders in patients evaluated for bariatric surgery. *Obes Surg*. 2003;13(5):676-683.
7. Schug SA, Raymann A. Postoperative pain management of the obese patient. *Best Pract Res Clin Anaesthesiol*. 2011;25(1):73-81.
8. Ahmad S, Nagle A, McCarthy RJ, Fitzgerald PC, Sullivan JT, Prystowsky J. Postoperative hypoxemia in morbidly obese patients with and without obstructive sleep apnea undergoing laparoscopic bariatric surgery. *Anesth Analg*. 2008;107(1):138-143.
9. Grover BT, Priem DM, Mathiason MA, Kallies KJ, Thompson GP, Kothari SN. Intensive care unit stay not required for patients with obstructive sleep apnea after laparoscopic Roux-en-Y gastric bypass. *Surg Obes Relat Dis*. 2010;6(2):165-170.
10. Batistich S, Kendall A, Somers S. Analgesic requirements in morbidly obese patients. *Anaesthesia*. 2004;59(5):510-511.
11. Charghi R, Backman S, Christou N, Rouah F, Schricker T. Patient controlled i.v. analgesia is an acceptable pain management strategy in morbidly obese patients undergoing gastric bypass surgery. A retrospective comparison with epidural analgesia. *Can J Anaesth*. 2003;50(7):672-678.

12. Lang SA, Arraf J. Analgesia in bariatric patients following upper abdominal surgery. *Can J Anaesth*. 2004;51(3):276; author reply 276.

13. Schug SA. The role of COX-2 inhibitors in the treatment of postoperative pain. *J Cardiovasc Pharmacol*. 2006;47(suppl 1):S82-S86.

14. Abernethy DR, Greenblatt DJ. Drug disposition in obese humans. An update. *Clin Pharmacokinet*. 1986;11(3):199-213.

15. Remy C, Marret E, Bonnet F. State of the art of paracetamol in acute pain therapy. *Curr Opin Anaesthesiol*. 2006;19(5):562-565.

16. Corcoran GB, Wong BK. Obesity as a risk factor in drug-induced organ injury: increased liver and kidney damage by acetaminophen in the obese overfed rat. *J Pharmacol Exp Ther*. 1987;241(3):921-927.

17. Schenker S, Speeg KV Jr, Perez A, Finch J. The effects of food restriction in man on hepatic metabolism of acetaminophen. *Clin Nutr*. 2001;20(2):145-150.

18. Blake DW, Yew CY, Donnan GB, Williams DL. Postoperative analgesia and respiratory events in patients with symptoms of obstructive sleep apnoea. *Anaesth Intensive Care*. 2009;37(5):720-725.

19. Choi YK, Brolin RE, Wagner BK, Chou S, Etesham S, Pollak P. Efficacy and safety of patient-controlled analgesia for morbidly obese patients following gastric bypass surgery. *Obes Surg*. 2000;10(2):154-159.

20. Etches RC. Respiratory depression associated with patient-controlled analgesia: a review of eight cases. *Can J Anaesth*. 1994;41(2):125-132.

21. Kyzer S, Ramadan E, Gersch M, Chaimoff C. Patient-controlled analgesia following vertical gastroplasty: a comparison with intramuscular narcotics. *Obes Surg*. 1995;5(1):18-21.

22. Levin A, Klein SL, Brolin RE, Pitchford DE. Patient-controlled analgesia for morbidly obese patients: an effective modality if used correctly. *Anesthesiology*. 1992;76(5):857-858.

23. VanDercar DH, Martinez AP, De Lisser EA. Sleep apnea syndromes: a potential contraindication for patient-controlled analgesia. *Anesthesiology*. 199;74(3):623-624.

24. Coldrey JC, Upton RN, Macintyre PE. Advances in analgesia in the older patient. *Best Pract Res Clin Anaesthesiol*. 2011;25(3): 367-378.

25. Monk TG, Weldon BC, Garvan CW, et al. Predictors of cognitive dysfunction after major noncardiac surgery. *Anesthesiology*. 2008;108(1):18-30.

26. Sinatra RS, Viscusi G, DeLeon-Cassasola O, Ginsberg B, eds. *Acute Pain Management*. London: Cambridge Press; 2009.

27. Drugs@FDA. Exparel Label and Approval History. US Food and Drug Administration web site. http://www.accessdata.fda.gov/scripts/cder/drugsatfda/index.cfm?fuseaction=Search.Label_ApprovalHistory. Published October 28, 2011. Accessed December 1, 2011.

28. Gagliese L, Gauthier LR, Macpherson AK, Jovellanos M, Chan VW. Correlates of postoperative pain and intravenous patient-controlled analgesia use in younger and older surgical patients. *Pain Med*. 2008;9(3):299-314.

29. Gagliese L, Katz J. Age differences in postoperative pain are scale dependent: a comparison of measures of pain intensity and quality in younger and older surgical patients. *Pain*. 2003;103(1-2):11-20.

30. Special Issue: Deaths related to opioids prescribed for chronic pain: causes and solutions. *Pain Med*. 2011;12(suppl 2):S13-S92.

16

Abbreviations/Acronyms

5-HT	5-hydroxytryptamine (serotonin)
AAPM	American Academy of Pain Medicine
AARP	American Association of Retired Persons
ADE	adverse drug event
AE	adverse event
AMP	α-amino3-hydroxy-5-methylisoxazole-4-proprionic acid
APAP	*N*-acetyl-para-aminophenol (acetaminophen)
ASA	American Society of Anesthesiologists
ASRA	American Society of Regional Anesthesia
ATP	adenosine triphosphate
AUC	area under the curve
BBB	blood-brain barrier
bid	twice a day
BK	bradykinin
Ca^{++}	calcium ion
CABG	coronary artery bypass graft
cAMP	cyclic adenosine monophosphate
CGRP	calcitonin gene-related peptide
CI	confidence interval
C_{max}	maximum concentration of drug
CMS	Center for Medicare and Medicaid Services
CNS	central nervous system
COX	cyclooxygenase
CR	controlled-release
CSF	cerebrospinal fluid
CV	cardiovascular
DVT	deep vein thrombosis
EAA	excitatory amino acid
ED	emergency department

EK	enkephalin
ENT	ear, nose, and throat
EPS	extra pyramidal symptoms
ER	extended release
EREM	extended-release epidural morphine
FDA	Food and Drug Administration
GABA	gamma-aminobutyric acid
GI	gastrointestinal
Glu	glutamate
h, hr	hour(s)
H^+	hydrogen ion
HCAHPS	Hospital Consumer Assessment of Healthcare Providers and Systems
IASP	International Association for the Study of Pain
ICU	intensive care unit
IL-1B	interleukin 1B
IM	intramuscular
IR	immediate release
IV	intravenous
JCAHO	Joint Commission on Accreditation of Healthcare Organizations
K^+	potassium ion
LA	local anesthetic
LC	locus caeruleus
LMWH	low molecular weight heparin
LOS	length of stay
MAC	monitored anesthesia care
MAOI	monoamine oxidase inhibitor
Mg^{++}	magnesium ion
mRNA	messenger ribonucleoprotein acid
NA	noradrenaline
Na^+	sodium ion
NE	norepinephrine
NK-1	neurokinin-1
NMDA	*N*-methyl-D-aspartate
NO	nitric oxide
NOS	nitric oxide synthase
NPO	nothing by mouth
NRM	nucleus raphes magnus
NS	nociceptive-specific

NSAID	nonsteroidal anti-inflammatory drug
nSTT	neospinothalamic tract
OIH	opioid-induced hyperalgesia
OSA	obstructive sleep apnea
OR	odds ratio
ORAE	opioid-related adverse event
$PaCO_2$	partial pressure (tension) of carbon dioxide, artery
PACU	postanesthesia care unit
PAG	periaqueductal gray
PBO	placebo
PCA	patient-controlled analgesia
PCEA	patient-controlled epidural analgesia
PG	prostaglandin
PKA	phosphokinase-A
PNB	peripheral neural blockade
PO	by mouth (oral)
POD	postoperative delerium
POI	postoperative ileus
PRN	as needed
PROP	proparacetamol
pSTT	paleospinothalamic tract
PVB	paravertebral block
qd	every day
qid	four times daily
RAS	reticular activating system
SAGES	Society of American Gastrointestinal and Endoscopic Surgeons
SC	subcutaneous
SF	short form
SNRI	serotonin-norephinephrine reuptake inhibitor
SP	substance P
SRE	system-related event
SSRI	selective serotonin reuptake inhibitor
STT	spinothalamic tract
TAH	total abdominal hysterectomy
TCA	tricyclic antidepressant
TEA	thoracic epidural anesthetic

TEAE	treatment-emergent adverse event
tid	three times a day
TKA	total knee arthroplasty
T_{max}	time of occurrence for maximum (peak) drug concentration
TNS	transient neurologic symptoms
TRP	tubular reabsorption of phosphate
TRPV-1	transient receptor potential voltage-one
VAS	visual analogue scale
VSR	visual rating scale
WDR	wide-dynamic range neurons

INDEX

Note: Page numbers in *italics* indicate figures.
Page numbers followed by a "t" indicate tables.

17

17

17

17

17